BASIC EKG INTERPRETATION

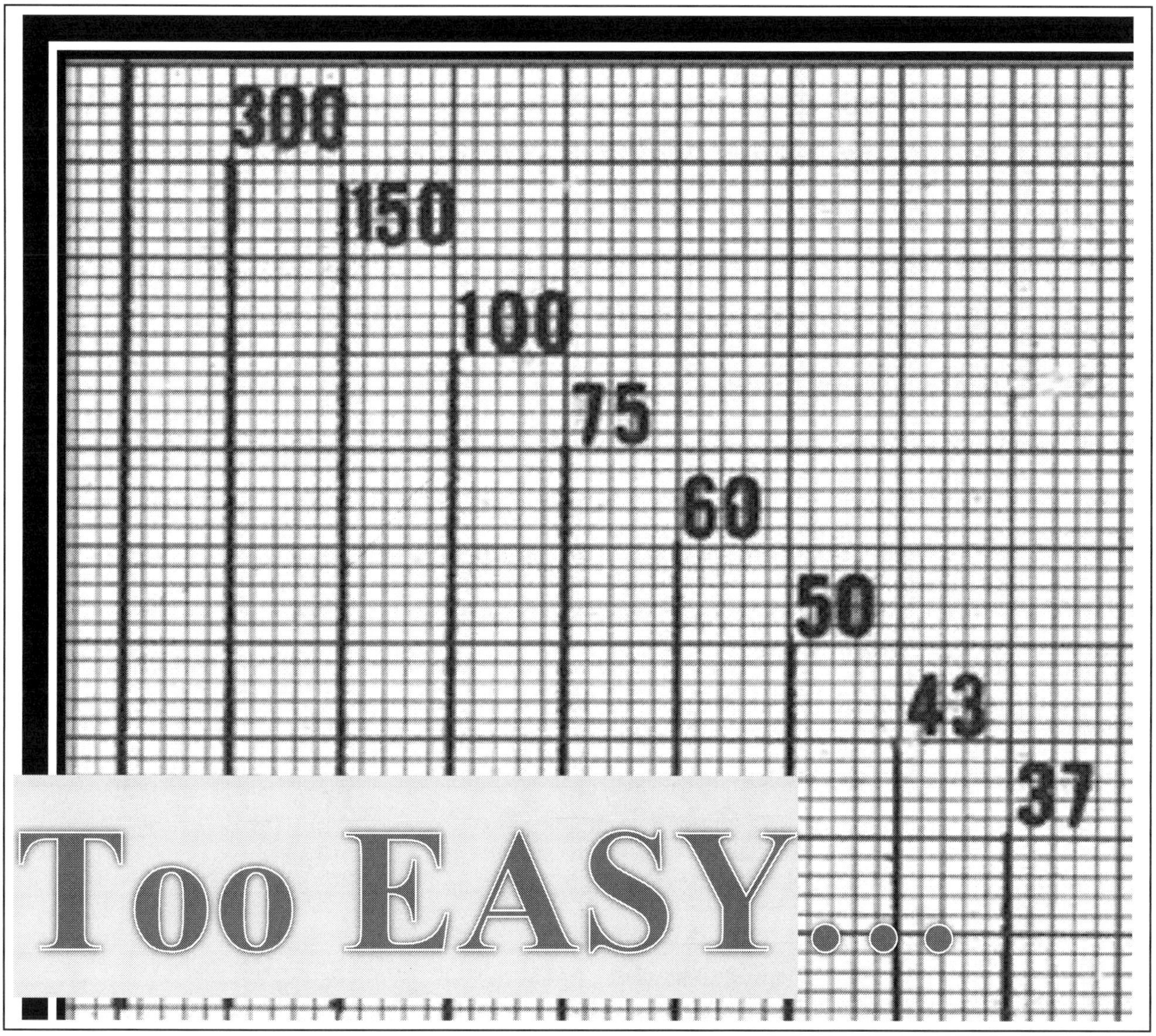

Too EASY...

-Medicsmith

"I can remember standing in the emergency center more than 25 years ago as an ER Tech and looking at the cardiac monitor totally lost in the rhythm. An old Army nurse asked me to tell her what I saw and with my best dumb look I gave her a confident shoulder shrug. Luckily for me she was not one to except that for an answer. For the next 2 years I sat at a desk watching cardiac monitors until I could diagnose cardiac rhythms by the sound of the beat. I owe her a lot."

• •

If EKG's are new to you all you see when you look at them right now is the Chevy symbol bouncing across the page. Well to you I say if you can keep time with a song you can read an EKG. I'm not going to teach in the same fashion as most books out there. It is not my intention to make you a cardiologist but to establish a foundation for you to build off of as you improve in the science of EKG interpretation.

To start, what do should we know about EKG interpretation? Take the time to remember the following points:

A. **An EKG is not a measurement of the hearts movement but the electricity that goes through the heart.**

B. **The paper an EKG is on is graph paper and every square, large and small relate to a measurement of time. ** each 1 mm (small) horizontal box corresponds to 0.04 second , with heavier lines forming larger boxes that include five small boxes and represent 0.20 sec.**

C. **The beat of the EKG should be equally spaced across the graph paper. Each cluster of bumps on the line should be the same distance from the next cluster of bumps.**

D. **If you pay attention to spacing you can qualify or disqualify many cardiac situations with the first glance at the monitor.**

Memorize these rules and you will quickly be able identify rhythms. Look at the picture of the graph paper below (pic A1). Across the top are small hash marks. The hash marks are 3 seconds away from each other.

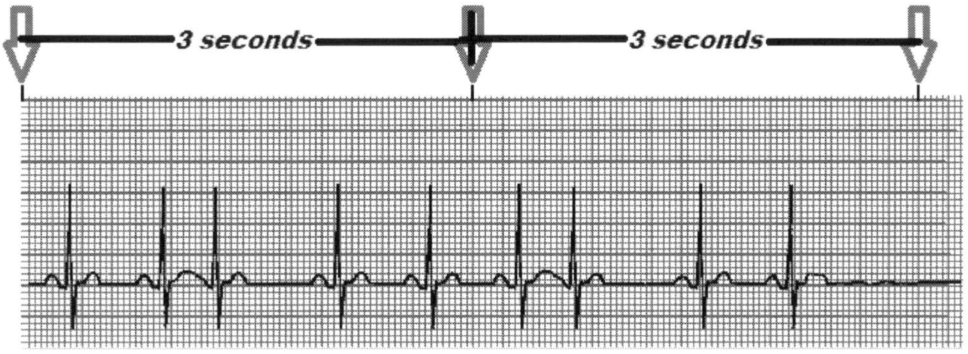

pic. A1

From time to time you may be asked for a “6 second strip”. This allows the physician or the medic to determine what is going on with the patient and approximately what the patient’s heart rate is over a one minute time frame.

So now that we understand what the paper is lets jump right into the first rhythm. The easiest rhythm to learn is the one rhythm that has no electrical activity to measure.

Remember the first rule we learned:

A. An EKG is not a measurement of the hearts movement but the electricity that goes through the heart.

Asystole

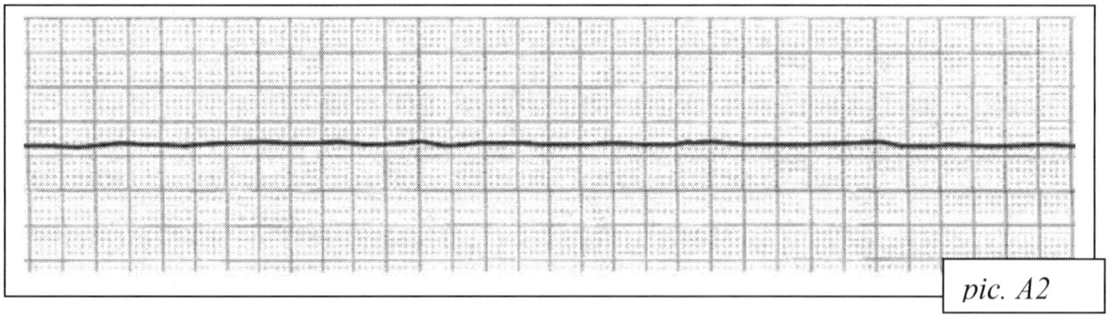

pic. A2

Asystole is the absence of all electrical activity in the heart muscle. Sometime called “Flat-Line” on TV and occasionally acted out being defibrillated. As will learn in later pages this rhythm is not shockable. For Asystole the patient is for all intensive purposes dead. However, should you see this on a cardiac monitor always check to verify all cardiac leads are in place and the patient is actually without a pulse. Many patients over the years have been injured by emergency staff that started compressions on a patient who had sweated off a lead.

Asystole: The absence of electrical activity in the heart muscle.

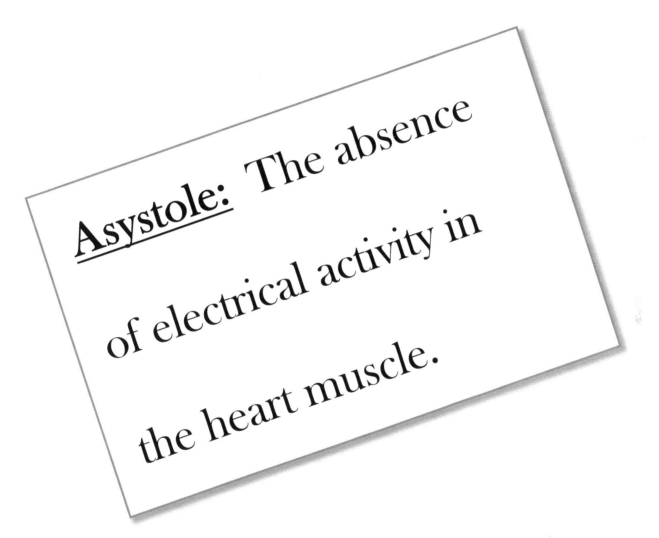

Activity: Draw Asystole on a piece of paper; a six second strip.

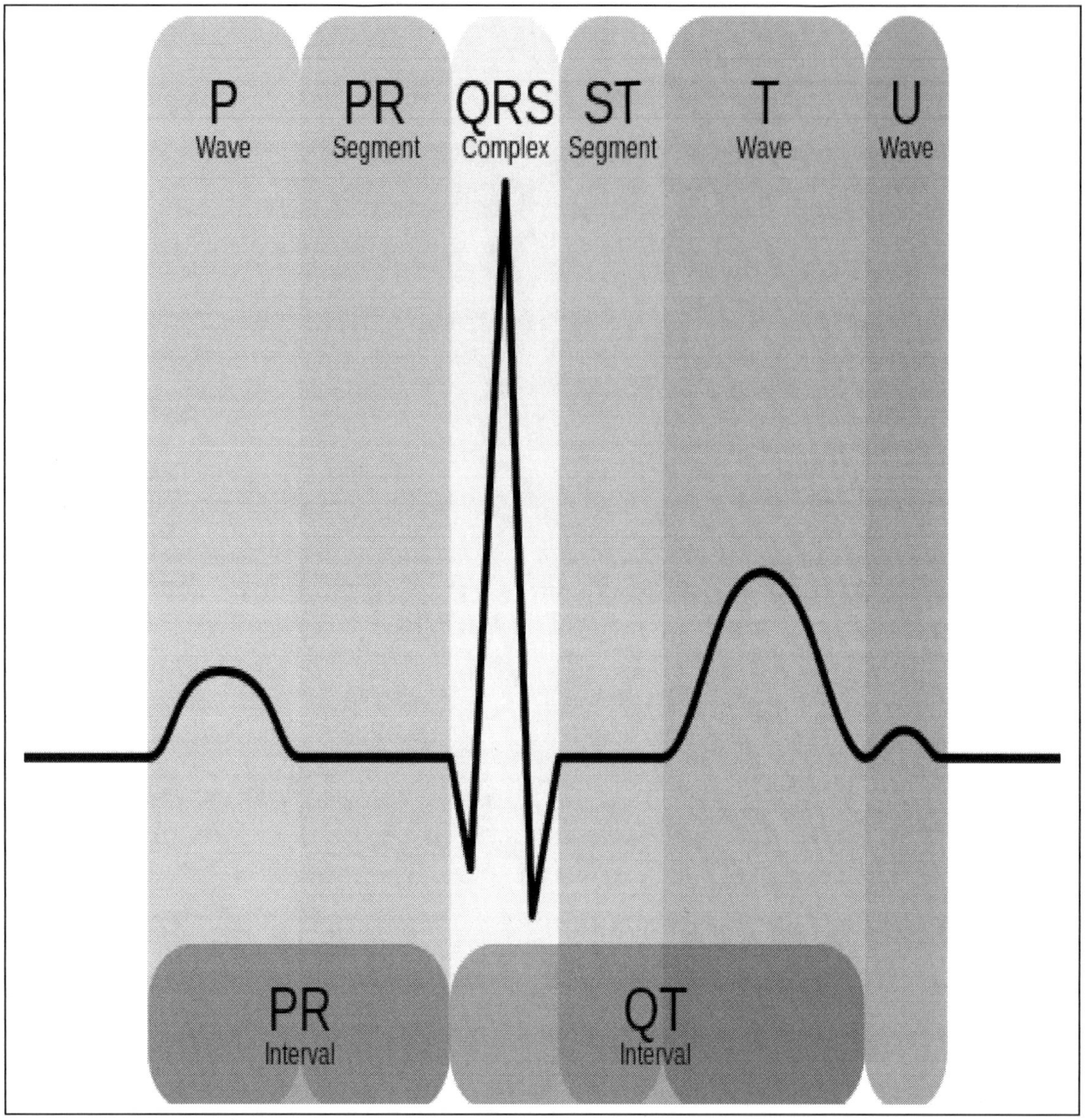

So each bump in the cluster has a corresponding label assigned to it that has significance to identification. What some folks get hung up on is how the bumps were named. Here is the quick and simple answer: when the bumps or "inflections" or "waves" were named the author started with the first letter in the alphabet that was not already assigned to something. Ergo “P” was the available character to be utilized.

The P wave:

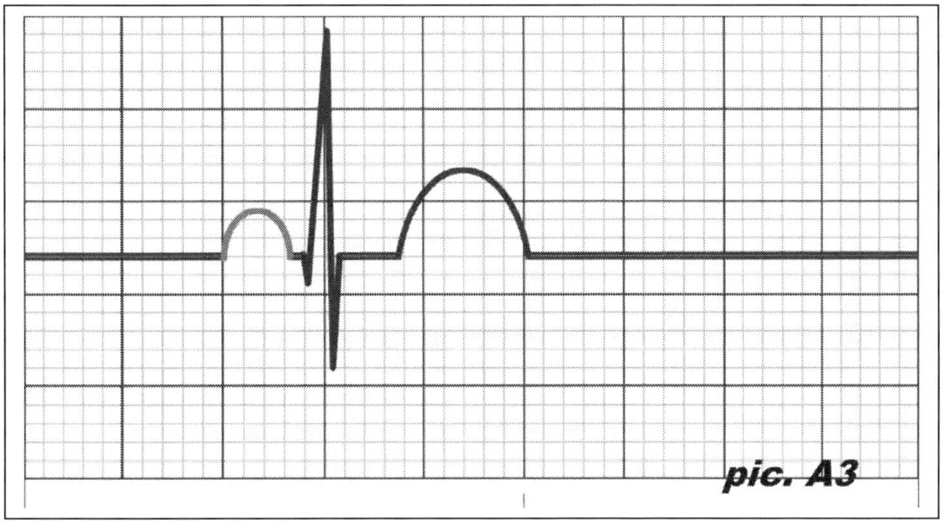

pic. A3

When the atrium contracts, which is known as DEPOLARIZATION, there is an upward inflection on the base line (the line in which all of the waves originate from).

The “P” wave is usually semi-lunar in shape and should always be in a cluster with the “RS” complex.

There should be no more than 3 small boxes between the “P” wave and the “QRS” complex. It is important to remember this is a TRANSLATION OF TIME recorded on graph paper. Therefore the time related between the “P” wave and next movement on the baseline should be around .12 seconds. In no time you will begin to measure the area with your eyes and anything bigger than 3 small boxes will jump out at you.

I once had a teacher that described the cluster of waves in the cardiac cycle as a gun being fired. The “P” wave represents the hammer being pulled back. The resulting “QRS” complex would be the bullet leaving the gun.

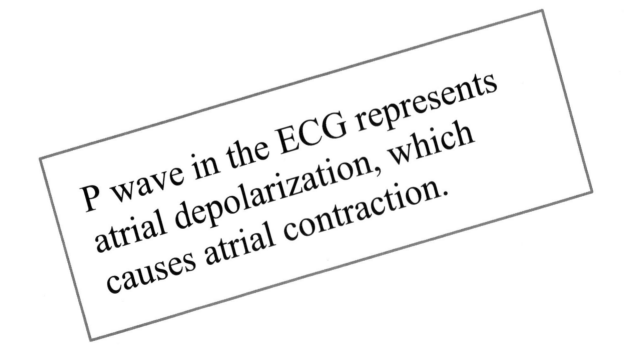

P wave in the ECG represents atrial depolarization, which causes atrial contraction.

<u>The Q wave:</u>

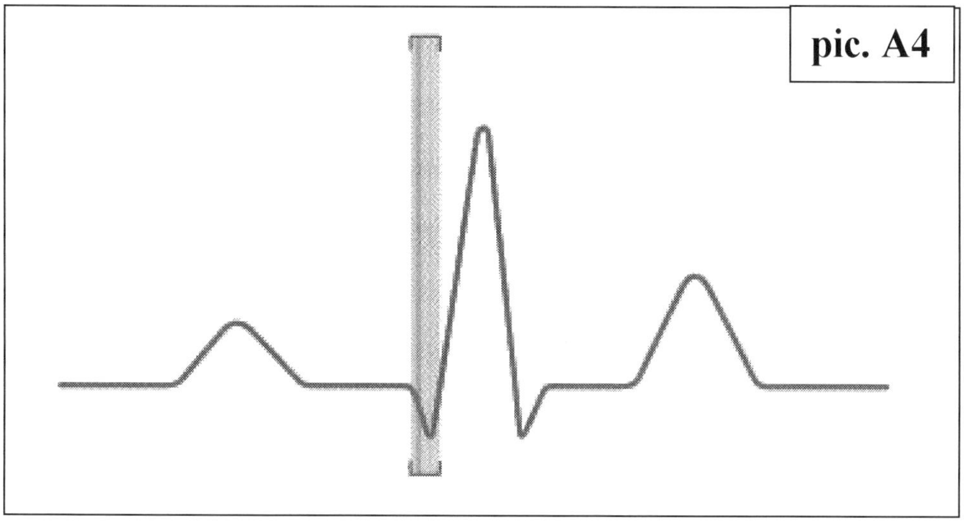

pic. A4

The “Q” wave is the negative or downward deflection from the baseline immediately before the “RS” waves in the cluster. There is a small amount of depolarization that happens in the septum of the heart which is captured in this wave. Back to our analogy of firing the gun the “Q” wave would be the action of squeezing the trigger. Therefore the “Q” wave is small and should never be greater than 2 small boxes. If it is however, it must be compared the “RS” waves. If the “Q” wave is greater than 2/3’s the size of the “RS” wave you will most likely be witnessing a patient which is having an Acute Myocardial Infarction (AMI).

The “Q” may be a positive movement from the baseline but only if the “RS” waves are in the opposite direction.

In some cardiac rhythms the “Q” wave may be virtually invisible. Don’t let that take too much of your attention. Remember that it only should capture a small amount of electrical activity on the septum of the heart so it can be very small or absent.

If the “Q” wave is greater than 2/3’s the size of the “RS” wave you will most likely be witnessing a patient which is having an Acute Myocardial Infarction (AMI).

<u>The QRS complex:</u>

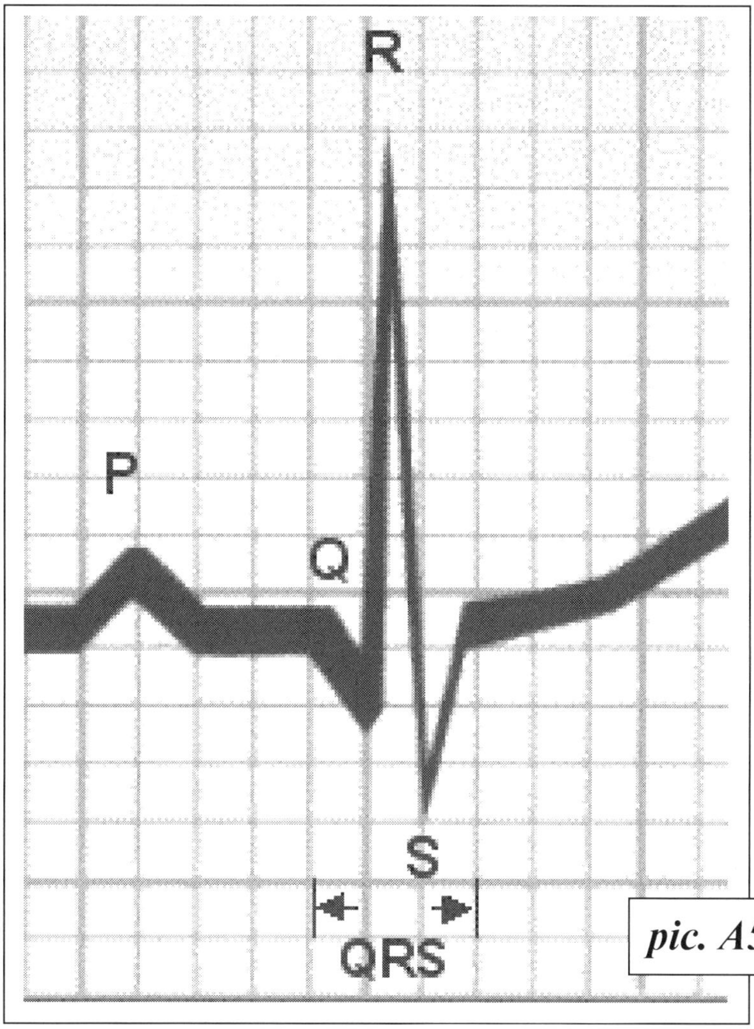

pic. A5

The "QRS" complex is the meat of the cardiac cycle. This powerful contraction of the Right & Left Ventricle is what really makes the entire cycle work. In our gun analogy this is the bullet leaving the barrel. The "QRS" complex is a combination of the three respective waves and should be narrow in nature; usually between .06-1.0 seconds (between 1 to less than 3 small boxes).

As this group of waves is so powerful it is paramount in not only the interpretation of an EKG but the source of life itself. Though many components must happen in time to make the heart beat effectively if the "QRS" complex malfunctions life may not be sustainable.

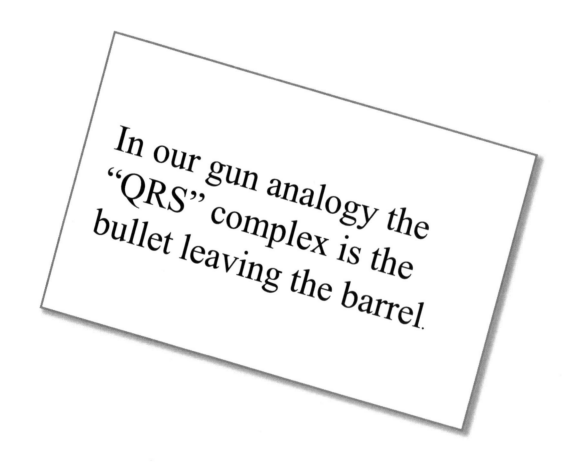

> In our gun analogy the "QRS" complex is the bullet leaving the barrel.

The T complex:

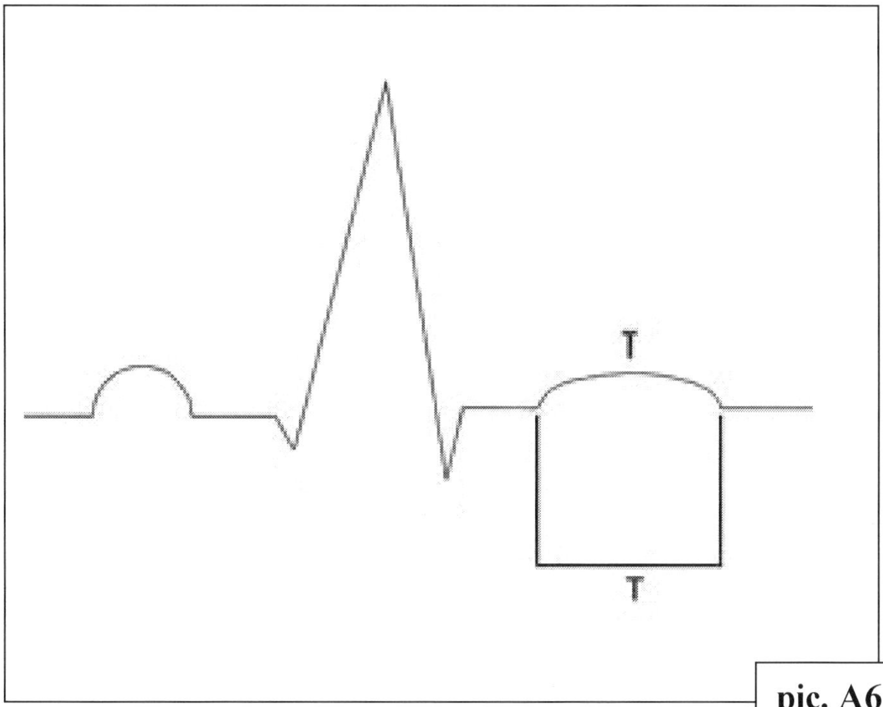

pic. A6

The “T” wave signifies the rest period or refractory (recovery) of the ventricles. This wave should be a little flatter than the “P” wave and should also be a little wider. It is important to note the “T” wave is an important indicator in the recognition of many cardiac abnormalities as well as ischemia or lack of oxygen to the cardiac tissue.

The EKG tracing:

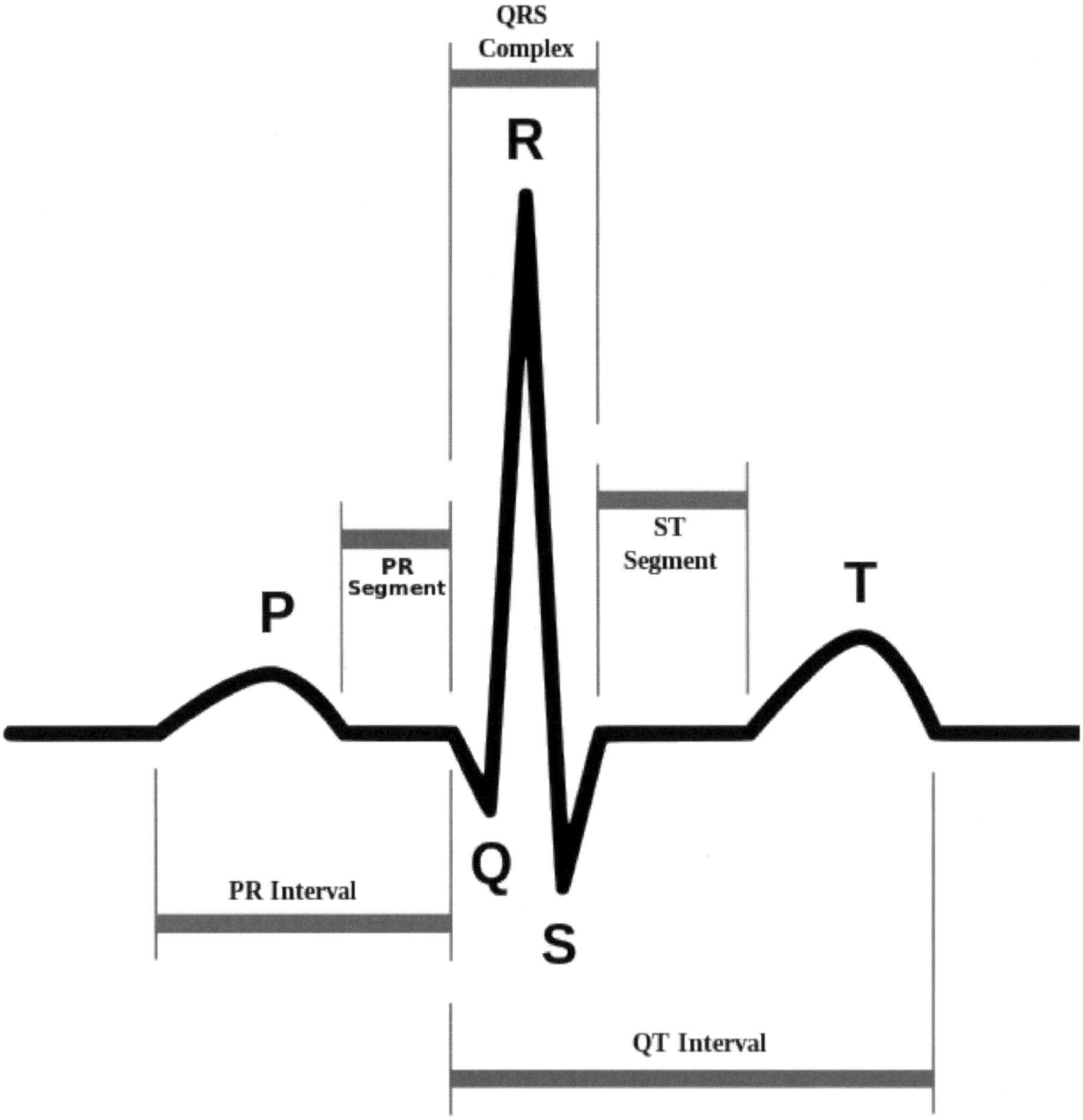

pic. A7

Activity: On this page draw all the waves in sequence. Remember proper spacing of the individual waves.

Cardiac Conduction System

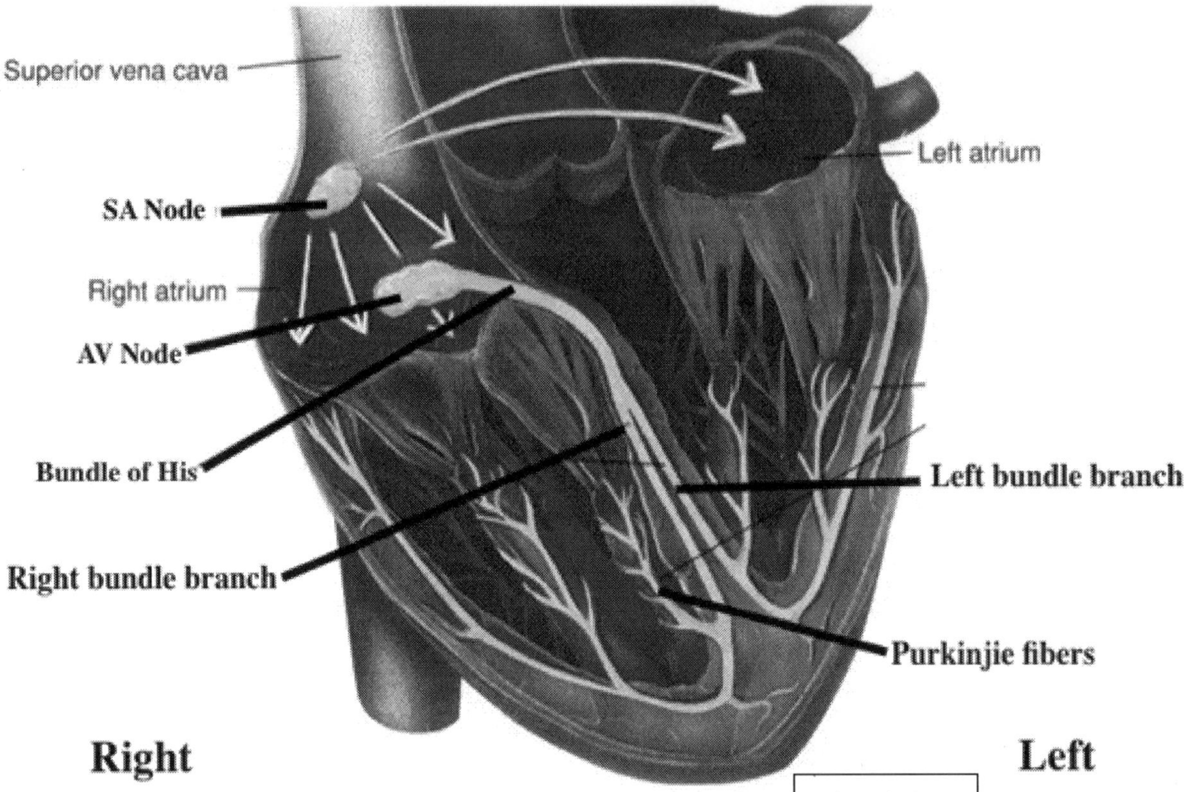

pic. A8

As mentioned earlier the EKG measures not Cardiac motion but the electrical activity the passes through the heart during the cardiac cycle. The electrical wave causes contraction in the muscle of the heart which in turn forces blood through the chambers of the heart, into the lungs, back into the heart, out to the body, then returns to the heart to begin all over again. For the purpose of this first manual we are only concerned which the electrical activity and not as much with the physiology of the muscle. In the upper left hand corner of this picture of the heart is the SA Node which is actually the upper right side of the heart. **The SA Node or Sinoatrial Node is the pacemaker for the heart. When the SA Node is functioning properly the rate of the heart will be at 60-80 beats per minute in a healthy resting heart.**

Past the SA Node is the AV Node or Atrioventricular (AV) Node. This cluster of cells receives signals from the SA Node sends signals from the atria to the ventricles once it has been reduced and synchronized. The AV Node is important in that it allows the atria time to empty before closing, thus preventing regurgitation of blood backwards in the circulatory system.

If the SA Node fails the AV Node will take its place. However, the rate of the AV Node is much slower and will have a rate of 40-60 beats per minute.

The impulse initiated in the SA Node travels down the heart through the Bundle of His. Then splitting into the Left and Right Bundle Braches and finally terminating in the Purkinje Fibers. The muscle of the heart contracts and the impulse passes through.

This electrical path has been described as Christmas tree lights, blinking in sequence creating a beautiful display. Should a single light along the chain burn out or fail the lights further down the line will be affected. The electrical pathway of the heart works in a similar fashion.

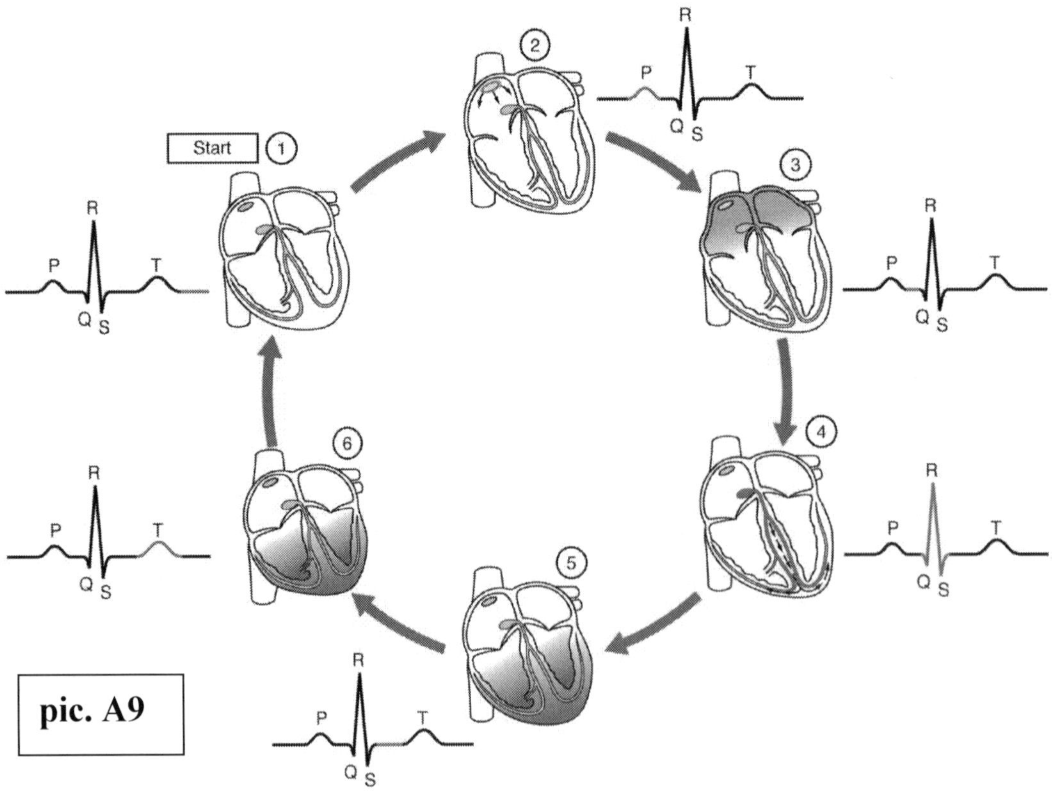

pic. A9

Counting Rate

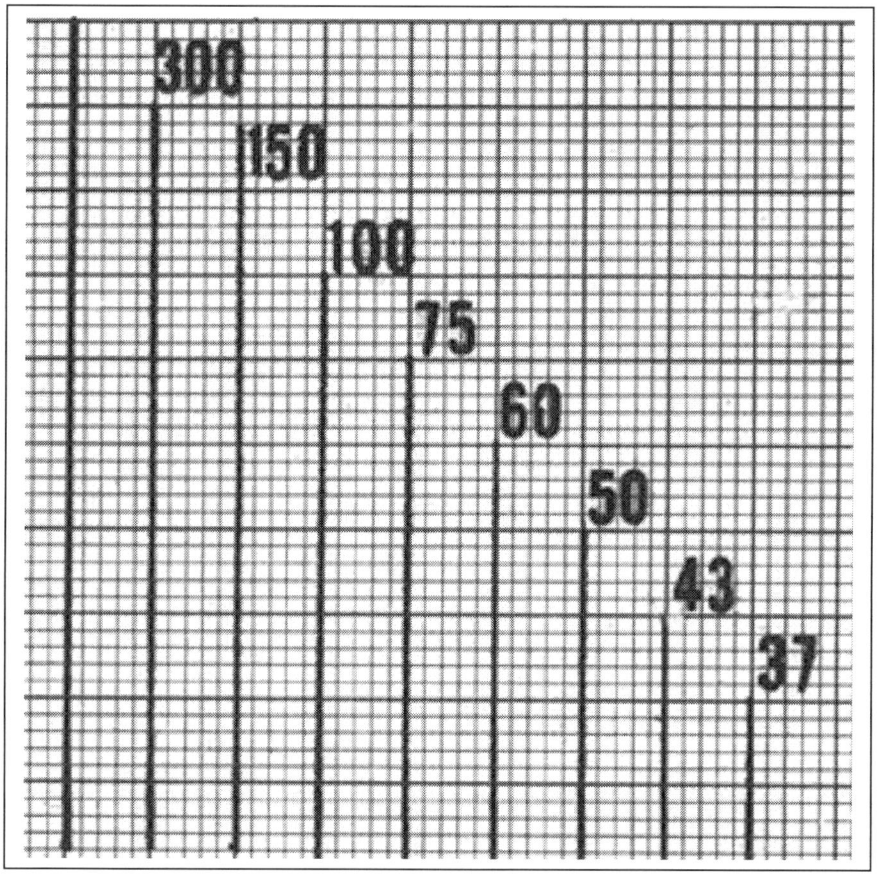

There are many schools of thought on how to determine the rate on an EKG strip. The only really important factor is that you can do it rapidly and without error. On the previous page is a tried and true method of counting the large boxes back from 300 from one “QRS” complex to the next “QRS” complex. My only complaint in this process is if you can’t remember how the numbers go….300..150..100..75..60..50..43..37..etc, you are going to lose valuable time with your patient. So I recommend just keeping it simple.

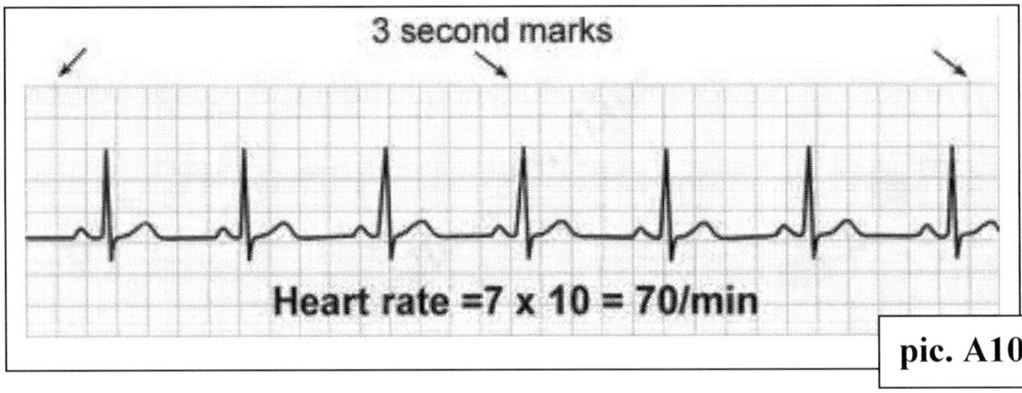

pic. A10

The illustration above shows the easiest and fastest way to get a heart rate. Earlier we discussed the hash marks on the top of the EKG strips. These marks are placed every 3 seconds. On a 6 second strip or 3 hash marks you simply count how many “QRS” complexes fall between the 1st and 3rd hash mark. Start as close to the first hash mark and end as close as possible to the last hash mark. Multiply this number by 10 and that gives you how many heart beats per minute that you have.

On the following examples practice your skills.

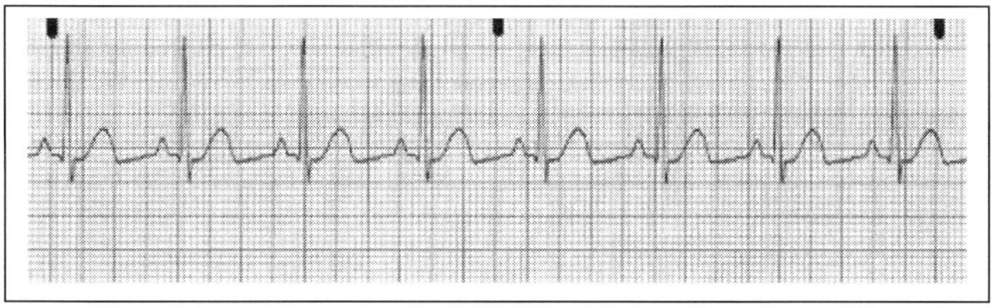

1. __________ BPM

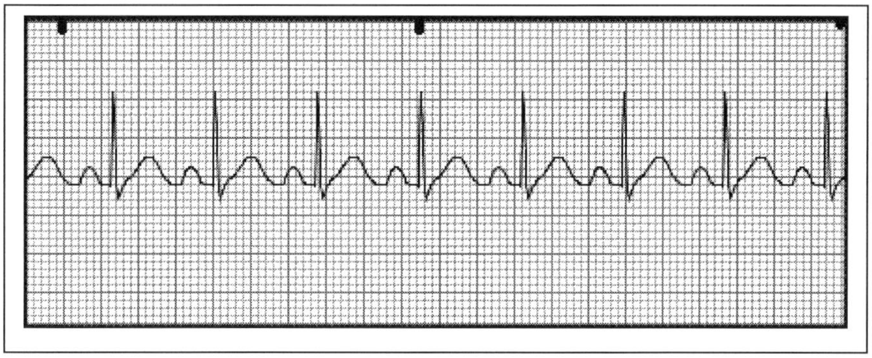

2. __________BPM

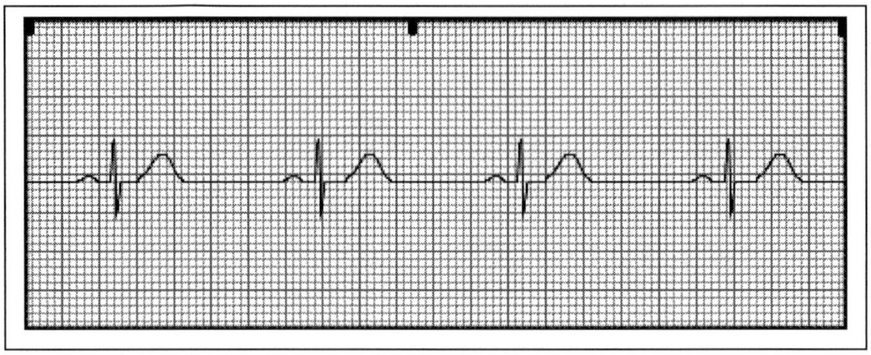

3. ___________BPM

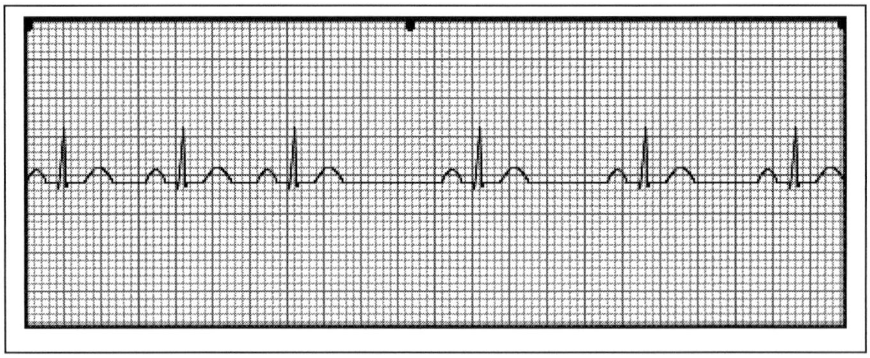

4. ___________BPM

1. 80 BPM 2. 90 BPM 3. 45-50 BPM 4. 60-65 BPM

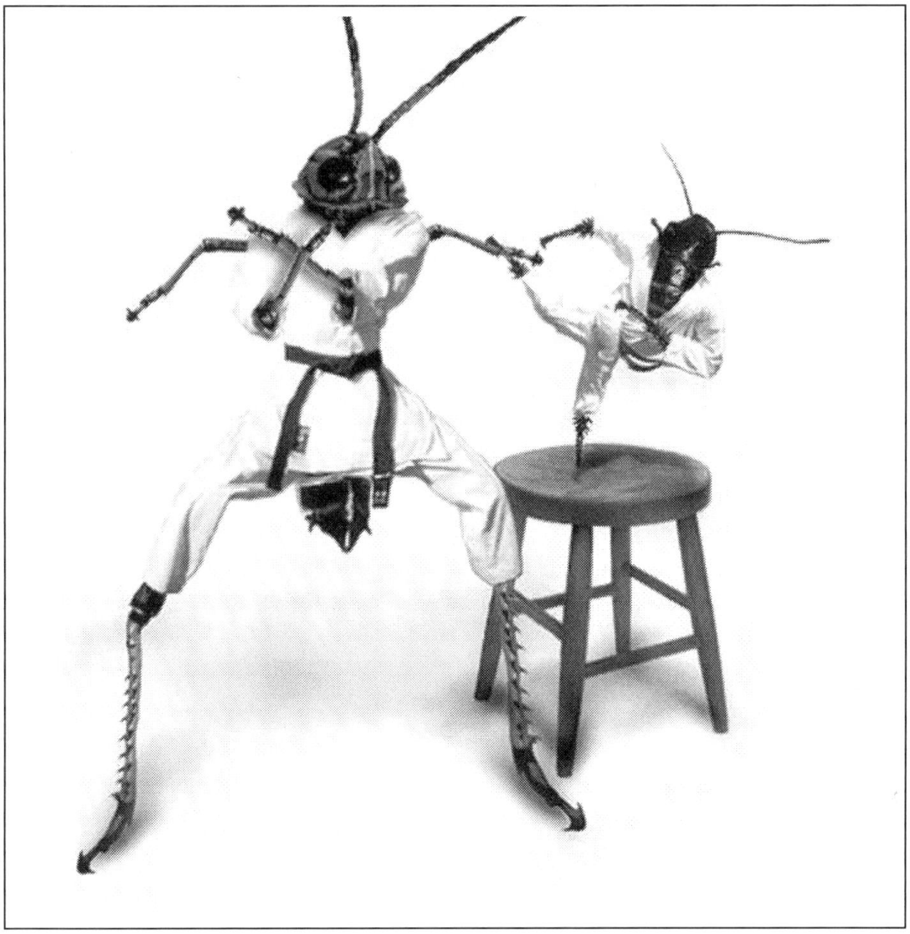

PUTTIN' IT ALL TOGETHER…

Now we understand rate, conduction, and the waves we can start identifying rhythms. Below are some of the rhythms we will be viewing:

1. NORMAL SINUS RHYTHM
2. SINUS BRADYCARDIA
3. SINUS TACHYCARDIA
4. SUPERVENTRICULAR TACHYCARDIA (SVT)
5. VENTRICULAR TACHYCARDIA (VTACH)
   A. WIDE
   B. NARROW
6. JUNCTIONAL RHYTHM
7. IDIOVENTRICULAR RHYTHM
8. 1ST DEGREE AV BLOCK
9. 2ND DEGREE AV BLOCK
10. 3RD DEGREE AV BLOCK
11. PAC'S
12. PVC'S
13. 60 CYCLE INTERFERENCE
14. INTERFERENCE
15. STEMI

<u>INTRODUCTION & NEW RULES:</u>

A. EVERY COMPLEX SHOULD BE EQUALLY SPACED FROM EACH OTHER.

B. EVERY COMPLEX SHOULD HAVE A "P" WAVE.

C. EVERY COMPLEX SHOULD HAVE A "QRS" COMPLEX.

D. EVERY COMPLEX SHOULD HAVE A "T" WAVE.

E. ABSENCE OF ANY WAVE USUALLY SIGNIFIES A PROBLEM.

<u>3 RULES OF BLAME: IN ORDER-</u>

1. **<u>Blame Your Patient</u>**: this sounds off but if you have a patient with Asystole on the monitor who is talking to you, chances are high that they have either wiggled or sweated off an EKG lead; blame you patient. (DOESN'T MEAN TO GET RUDE.)
2. **<u>Blame Your Machine</u>**: the EKG machine is not the best indicator of your patient's condition. The machine can be wrong, look at your patient before making aggressive decisions that could have lasting effects on your patient.
3. **<u>Blame Yourself</u>**: If a patient on the monitor is showing signs of cardiac compromise and you have verified that all of the leads are

on and the machine is functioning properly, it is time for you to act quickly and competently.

Make a Guide:

To determine spacing and assure that the waves are equally spaced use a separate sheet of paper and make tic-marks to gauge waves.

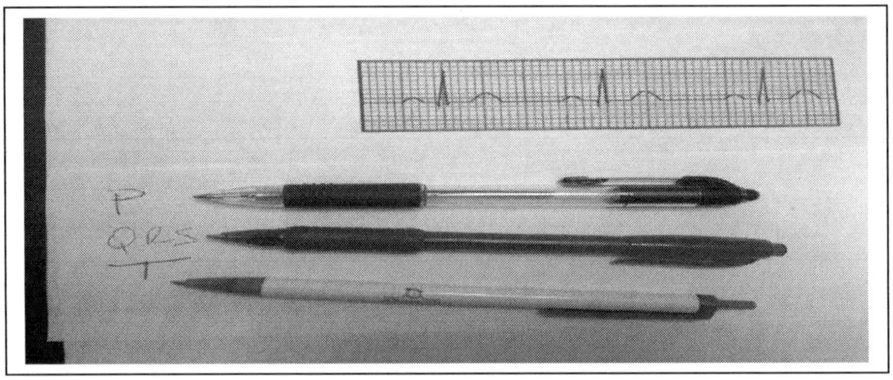

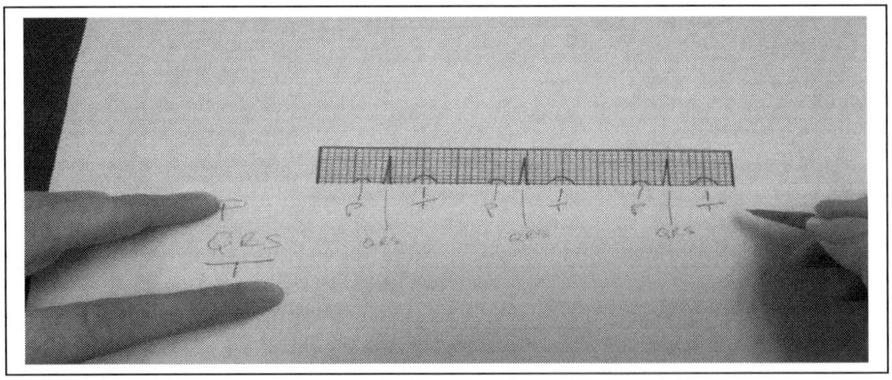

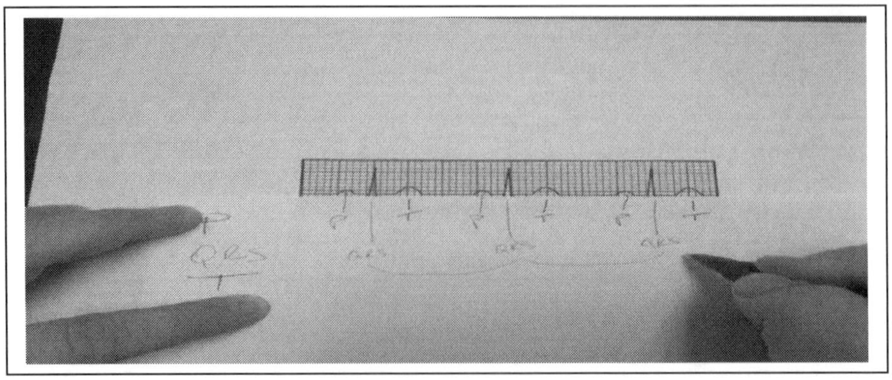

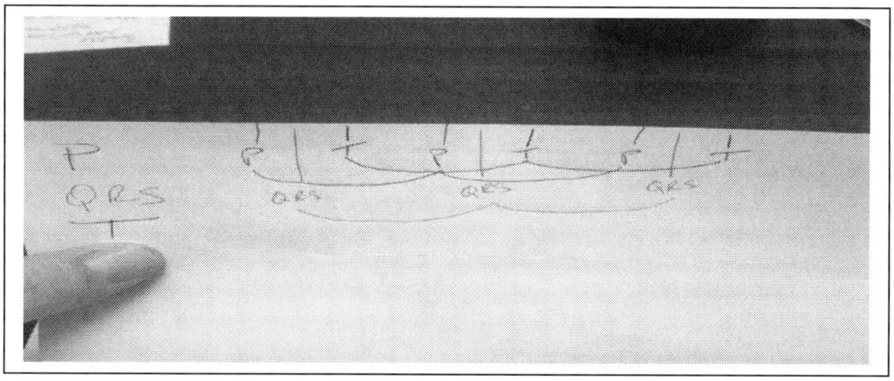

Using the "tic-marking system" check the following rhythms to see if they are regular:

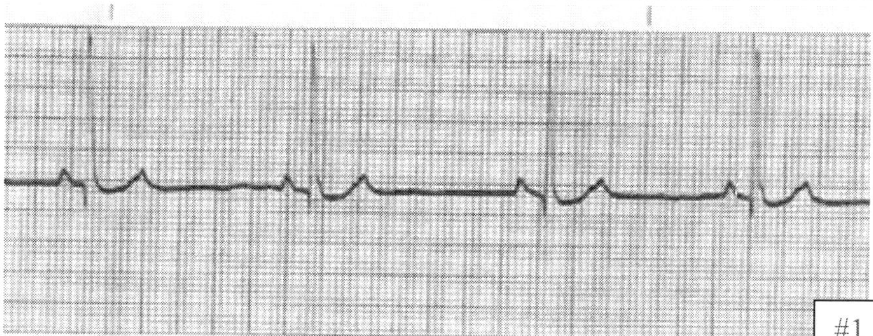

#1

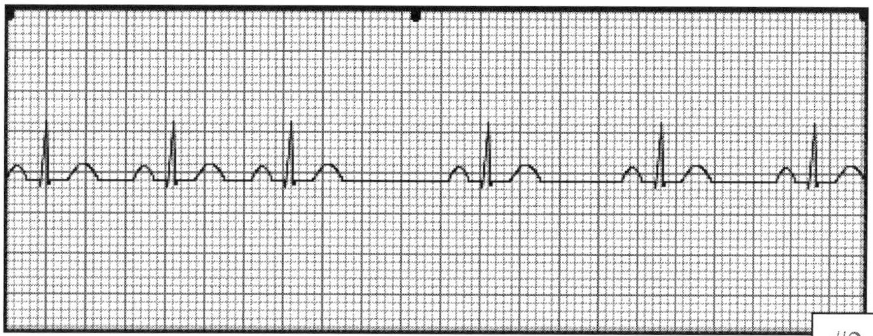

#2

#1 is Regular or Normal. #2 is Irregular.

Normal Sinus Rhythm (NSR)

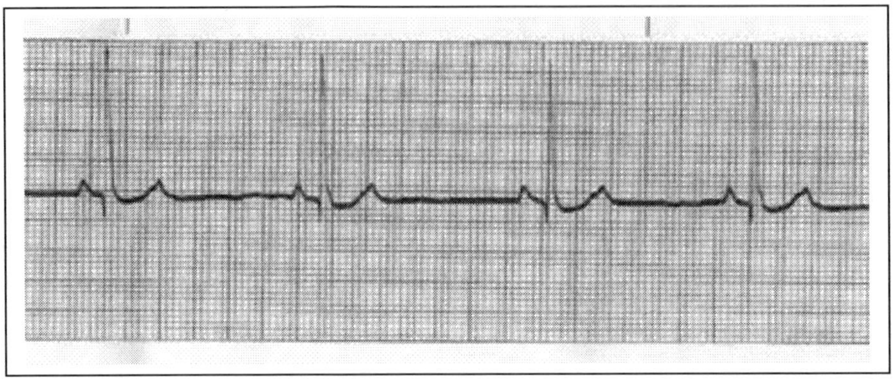

Questions to ask:

1. Is there a P wave for every QRS complex? ________________
2. Is there a T wave for every QRS complex? ________________
3. Is the rate greater than 60 but less than 90? ________________
4. Are there any abnormal waves? ________________________
5. Draw NSR in the space below:

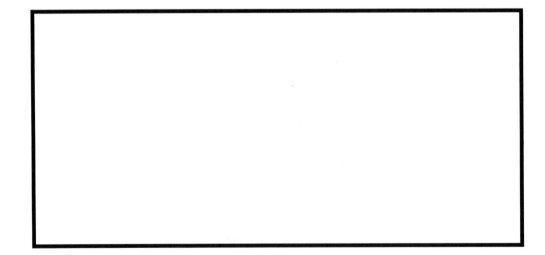

Sinus Bradycardia (Brady)

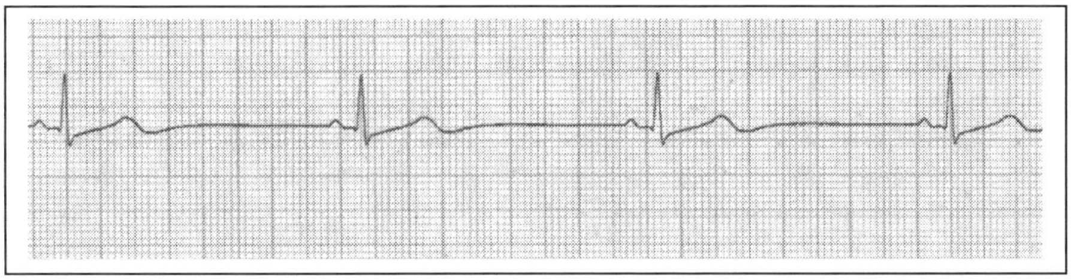

Questions to ask:

1. Is there a P wave for every QRS complex? ________________
2. Is there a T wave for every QRS complex? ________________
3. Is the rate greater than 60 but less than 90? ________________
4. Are there any abnormal waves? ________________________
5. Draw Sinus Bradycardia in the space below:

Sinus Tachycardia (Tach)

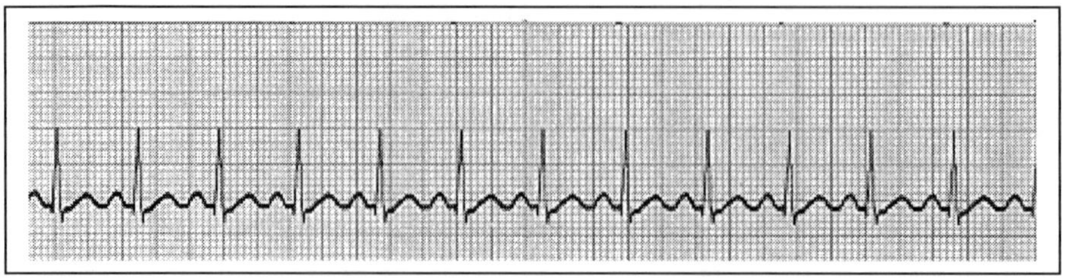

Questions to ask:

1. Is there a P wave for every QRS complex? _________________
2. Is there a T wave for every QRS complex? _________________
3. Is the rate greater than 60 but less than 90? _________________
4. Are there any abnormal waves? __________________________
5. Draw Sinus Tachycardia in the space below:

Super Ventricular Tachycardia (SVT)

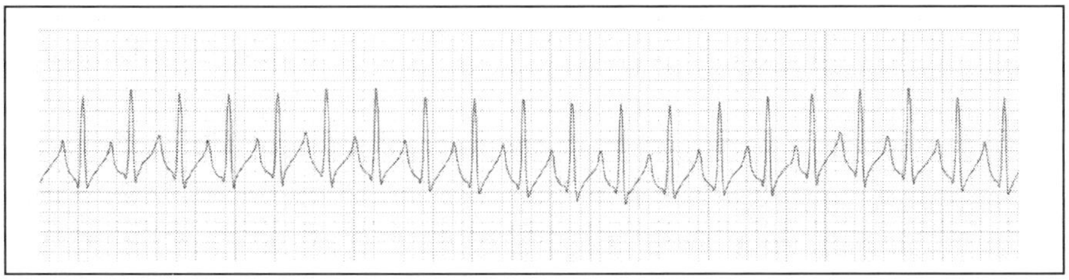

Questions to ask:

1. Is there a P wave for every QRS complex? ________________
2. Is there a T wave for every QRS complex? ________________
3. Is the rate greater than 60 but less than 90? ________________
4. Are there any abnormal waves? ________________________
5. Draw SVT in the space below:

Ventricular Tachycardia (VT)

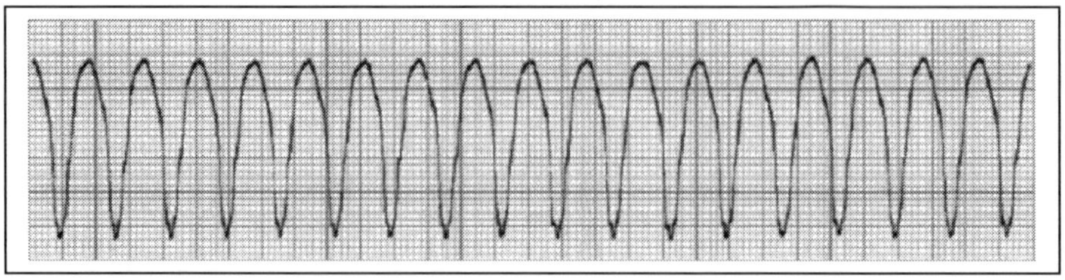

Questions to ask:

1. Is there a P wave for every QRS complex? ________________
2. Is there a T wave for every QRS complex? ________________
3. Is the rate greater than 60 but less than 90? ________________
4. Are there any abnormal waves? ________________________
5. Draw VT in the space below:

Ventricular Fibrillation (VFib)

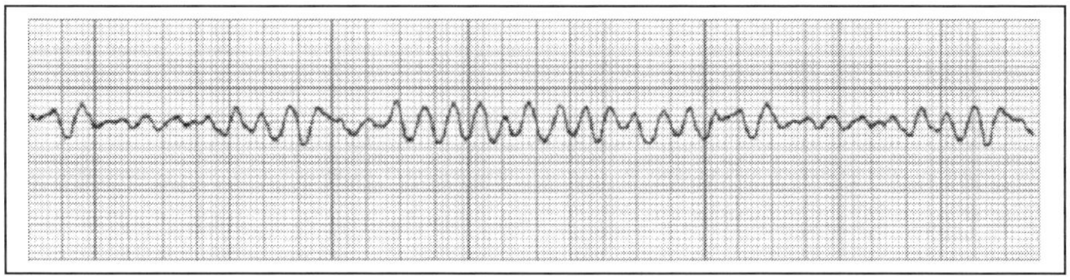

Questions to ask:

1. Is there a P wave for every QRS complex? ________________
2. Is there a T wave for every QRS complex? ________________
3. Is the rate greater than 60 but less than 90? ________________
4. Are there any abnormal waves? _________________________
5. Draw VFib in the space below:

Atrial Fibrillation (AFib)

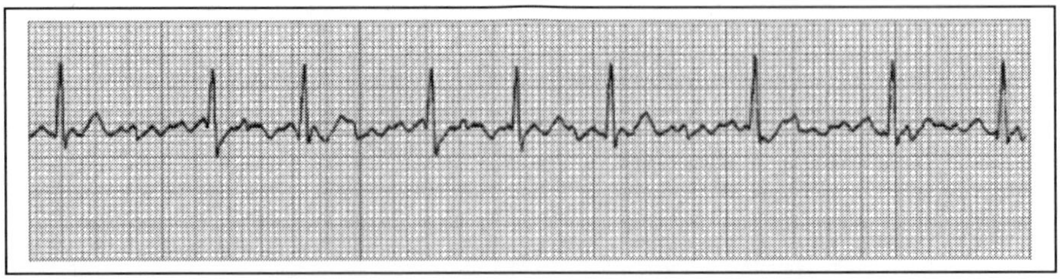

***Irregularly Irregular: may appear differently by always Irregular.

Questions to ask:

1. Is there a P wave for every QRS complex? ____________________
2. Is there a T wave for every QRS complex? ____________________
3. Is the rate greater than 60 but less than 90? ____________________
4. Are there any abnormal waves? ______________________________
5. Draw VFib in the space below:

Junctional Rhythm

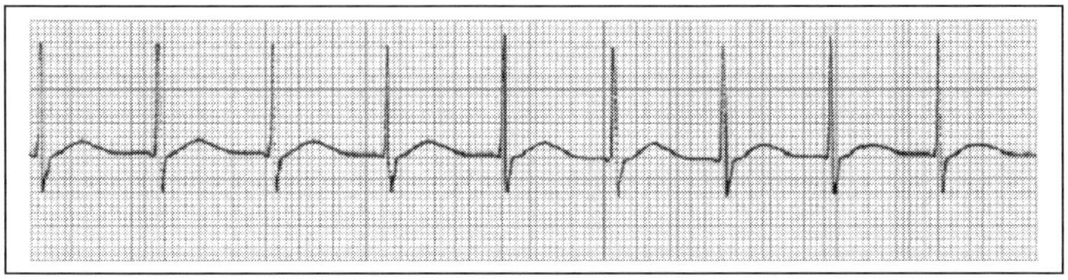

Questions to ask:

1. Is there a P wave for every QRS complex? ________________
2. Is there a T wave for every QRS complex? ________________
3. Is the rate greater than 60 but less than 90? ________________
4. Are there any abnormal waves? ________________________
5. Draw Junctional Rhythm in the space below:

Unifocal Premature Contraction (PVC)

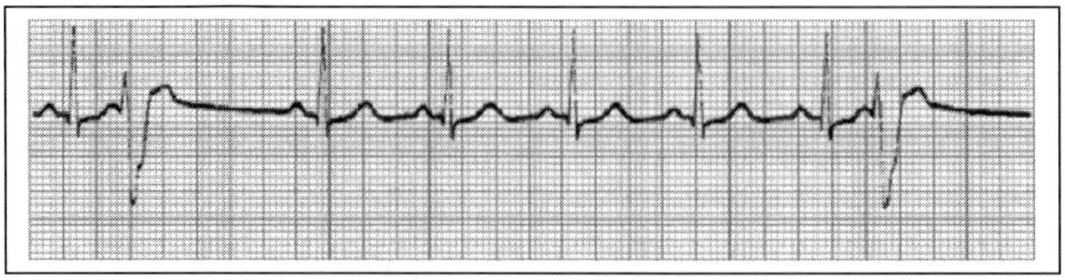

Questions to ask:

1. Is there a P wave for every QRS complex? ________________
2. Is there a T wave for every QRS complex? ________________
3. Is the rate greater than 60 but less than 90? ________________
4. Are there any abnormal waves? ________________________
5. Draw Unifocal PVC in the space below:

Monofocal Preventricular Contraction (PVC)

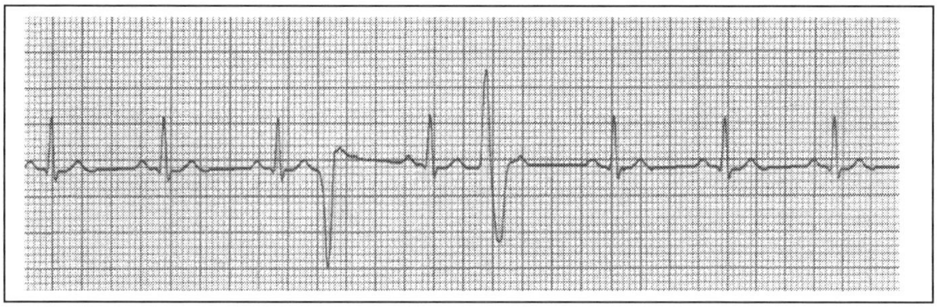

Questions to ask:

1. Is there a P wave for every QRS complex? ________________
2. Is there a T wave for every QRS complex? ________________
3. Is the rate greater than 60 but less than 90? ________________
4. Are there any abnormal waves? _________________________
5. Draw Monofocal PVC in the space below:

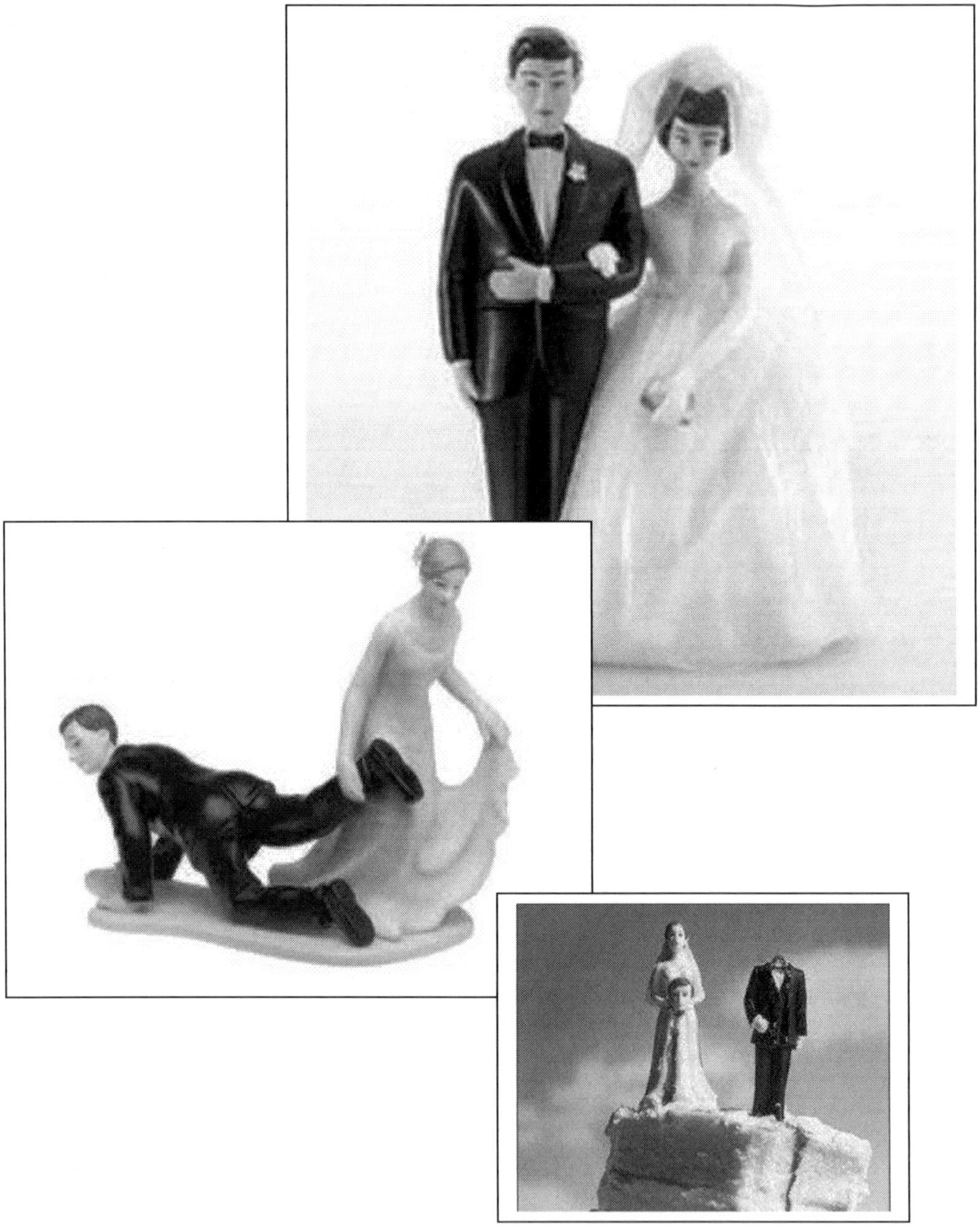

Heart Blocks

Heart Blocks have been the bane of existence to EMS and Hospital staff since the beginning of EKG recordings. "Is that Second Degree Heart block or is there a PAC, is this type one or type two, I know I look for a "P" wave but…uuuughhh!" To help you remember the things to look for I want to give you a simple analogy to put it all together.

Heart Blocks-The Marriage:

> **Remember to determine a Heart Block we look for the presence and position of the "P" wave in relationship to the "QRS" complex.

<u>Dating</u> – I can remember when I first met my wife, I couldn't get enough of her. To keep her name out of this lets just call her "P" and I was her big, strong "QRS". She didn't go anywhere without me and I felt that to be pretty normal. No complaints from my side.

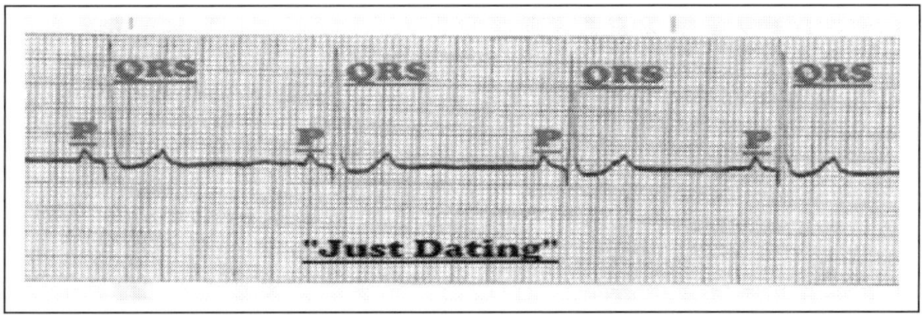

<u>Normal Sinus Rhythm.</u>

The FIRST YEAR:

So my beautiful girl "P" and I finally did it and tied the knot. The first year started off magical. The first 6 months or so we were inseparable. But like most relationships we were smothering each other. So by the end of the first year she pulled back a little. We were always together, me (QRS) and my girl (P) but she kept her own little space for herself always 2 steps or more behind me.

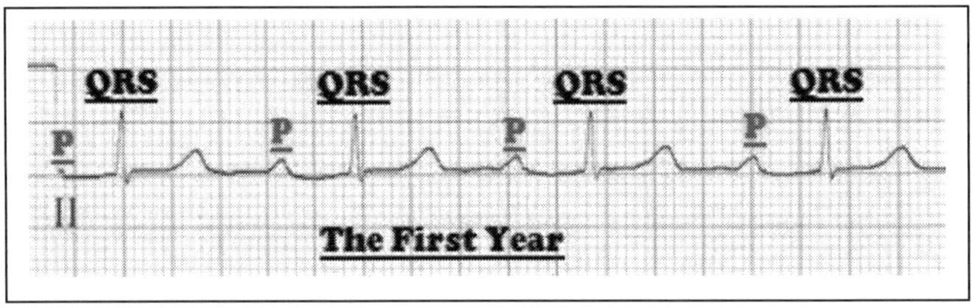

1st Degree AV Block

The SECOND YEAR: Hangin' In There

During our second year of marriage, me and P started picking up hobbies. I started going to baseball games and she would reluctantly go with me. Every Friday I had to rush her to get ready and each time she would take longer and longer to follow me out the door. Occasionally she would not go to the game with me at all. But she would feel bad and the whole cycle would start all over again.

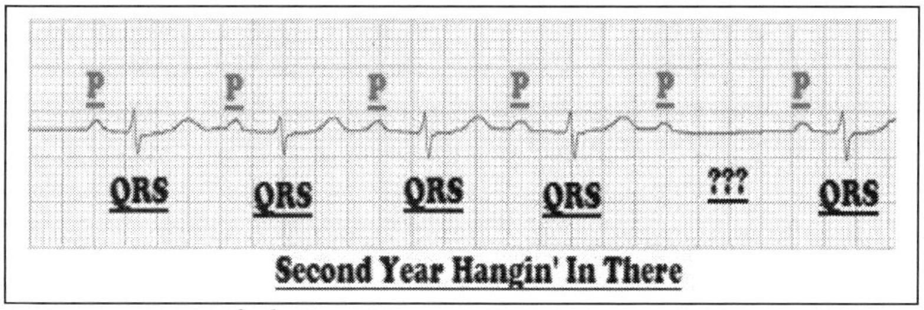

2nd Degree AV Block Type I

The SECOND YEAR: Gotta Go

To be fair with P, I agreed to start going to the mall and shopping. Guys if you haven't suffered through this it is complete H#**! I could make it with her a few times hand in hand but then I had to just bale and do my own thing for a day. But I would jump back into the cycle the next time.

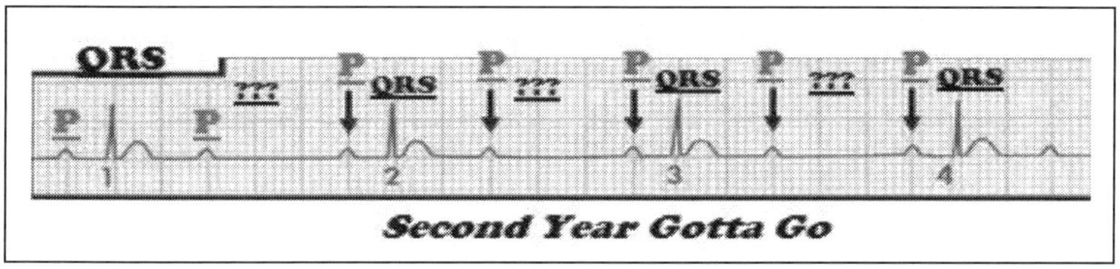

2nd Degree AV Block Type II

The SECOND YEAR: The Honey-moon is over!

Well Dad said that day would come. I can still hear him say, "Son behind every beautiful woman is a man tired of her crap." That is what happened to me and P in the third year. I had had enough of the mall and should would not step foot into a ball park. We became **complete**ly dysfunctional as a couple. I did my thing and she did hers. To be total honest we didn't get a lot accomplished in our **third** year.

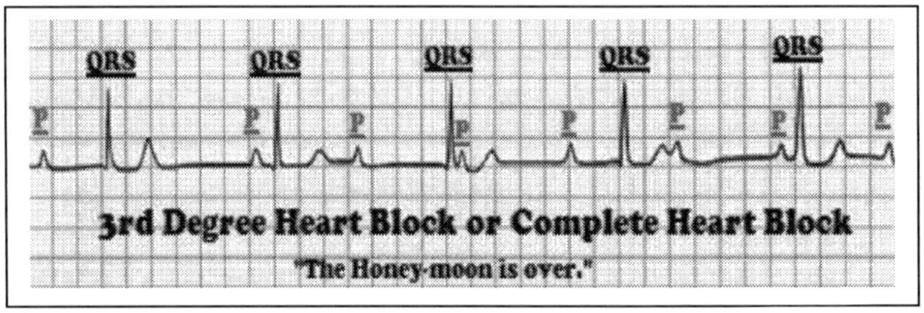

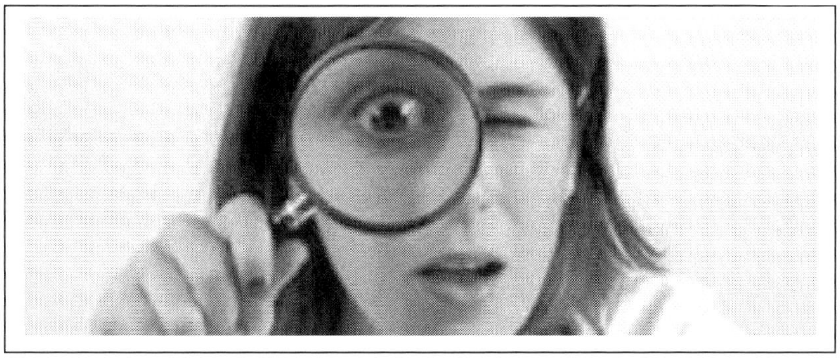

Rhythms to **LOOK** for…

╬ Atrial Fibrillation (AFib)

╬ Atrial Flutter

╬ Idioventricular

╬ Paced

╬ Ventricular Tachycardia (VTach)

╬ Ventricular Fibrillation (Vfib)

╬ Electrical Mechanical Disassociation (EMD)

- Also called Pulseless Electrical Activity (PEA)

The rhythms in this section have special features that must be recognized. In the above rhythms 3 are fatal if you do not intervene and the others can identify other underlying problems with your patient. The key is not to freak out and to follow the rules. We have already established that we look at the rhythm as a measurement of time. As we initially view the strip we look right away for the following:

1. Is the spacing of the “P-QRS-T” equal?
2. Is there a “P” wave for every “QRS” complex?
3. Is there a “T” wave for every “QRS” complex?

So with that in mind we will look at the next rhythms and apply the rules.

*** It should be said that whether or not the “QRS” is pointed up (positive), or down (negative) doesn’t really matter. Follow the rules and don’t get lost in the weeds.***

>>

╬ Atrial Fibrillation (AFib)

Rule: AFib is always “Irregularly Irregular” and the base line is sometimes referred to as “Noisy”. Additionally Afib is marked with an over generous amount of “P” waves. In this Rhythm the top and the bottom of the heart are not working well together. It has been noted that this condition is often related to Geriatric patients and those patients who have had a history of some type of stroke or TIA. Don't trust the heart rate on the monitor.

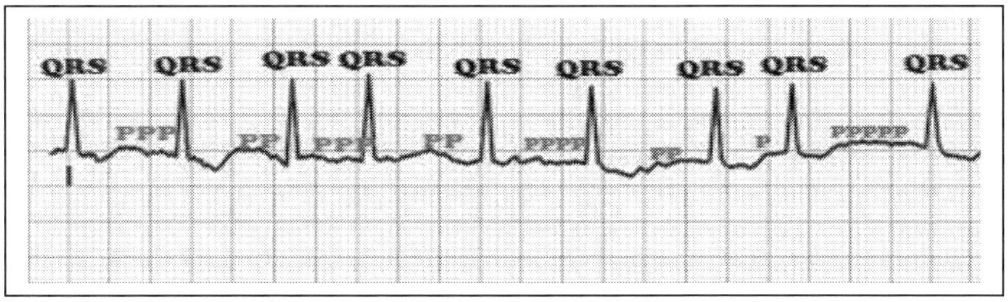

╬ Atrial Flutter

Atrial Flutter is a real problem. The atrial rate can be in or near the 300's, and with atrial dysrhythmias the "P" wave are everywhere. The actual Ventricular rate will be much slower. This patient is at great risk for clots forming and more vascular problems developing. The Atrial Flutter "P" wave is often referred to as "Saw-Toothed".

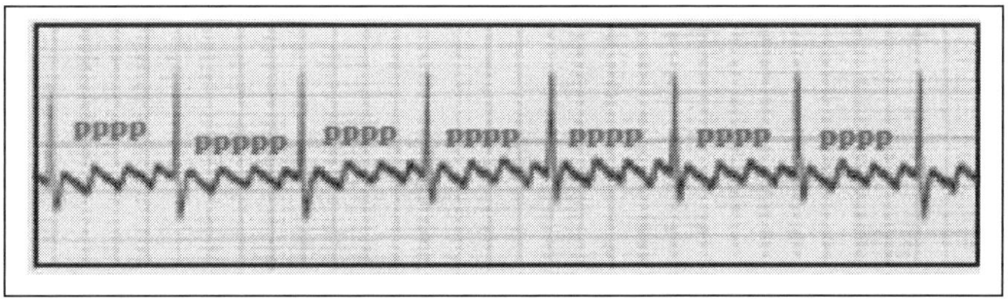

╬ Idioventricular

Idioventricular rhythms initiate not in the SA Node but from some Lone Ranger type cell from the ventricles. The rate will be much slower, 20-45 and there will be no “P” waves. The atrial part of the conduction system is not functioning appropriately.

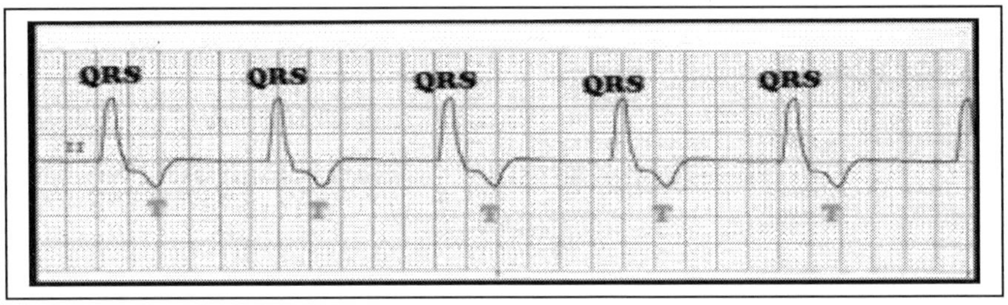

╬ Paced

Paced rhythms can be intimidating when you first see them; however once you learn to look for pacer spikes it will be less of an initial scare. Paced rhythms are just what they say, the pacer is firing and the cardiac monitor is recording the event. Watch your patient his condition and treat accordingly.

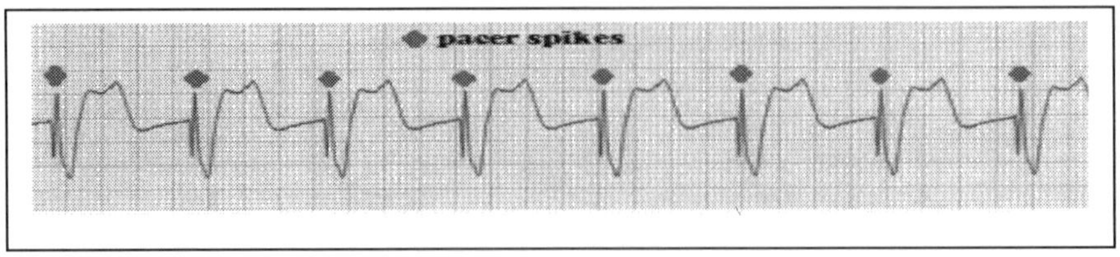

╬ Ventricular Tachycardia (VTach)

SHOCKABLE RHYTHM

VTach is a true medical emergency. If the rhythm becomes pulseless then it is one of the shockable rhythms that must be treated immediately. Follow you current ACLS guide for treatment standards. The diagnosis is made if 3 or more beats in a row, originating from the ventricles and will be more than 100 beats per minute. The rhythm may stop on its own but, for the most part, you will need to intervene. You must make every attempt to find the cause of the rhythm and treat according to your protocols.

Additionally the beats may be Wide or Narrow. There are specific treatment modalities for either Wide or Narrow complexes.

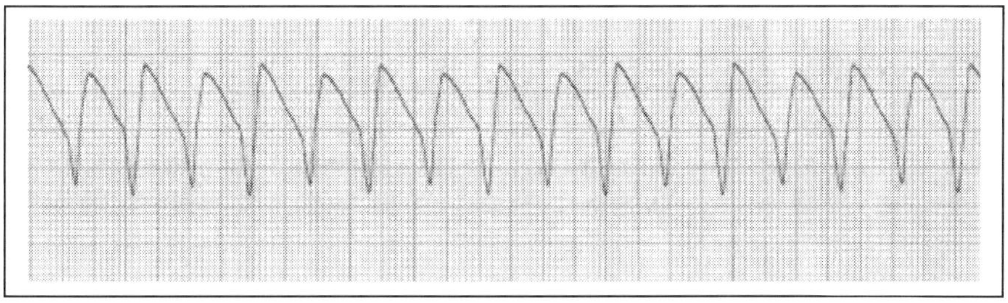

╬ Ventricular Fibrillation (VFib)

SHOCKABLE RHYTHM

VFib is THE MEDICAL EMERGENCY. The heart in this patient is in a fight with itself. Multiple foci in the heart are trying to fire at the same time, so instead of a heart beat the heat just quivers. If this continues for very much time at all the likelihood of the patient converting to Asystole is great. Start CPR, prepare tour cardiac monitor for defibrillation and follow ACLS guidelines.

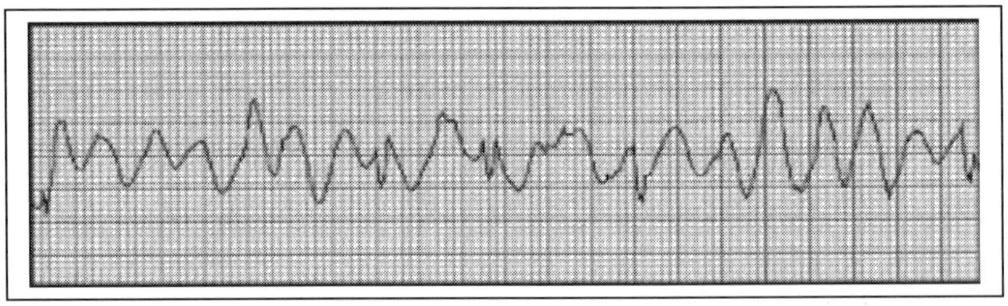

╬ Electrical Mechanical Disassociation (EMD)

Also called Pulseless Electrical Activity (PEA)

The Snake in the grass!

PEA is a condition in which the monitor displays a rhythm that may appear completely normal. However the patient will have no pulse and for all intensive purposes be dead. Remember the "3 Rule of Blame" from the front of this manual. When the patient doesn't look like what your equipment is telling you, assume your equipment is wrong and start assessing your patient.

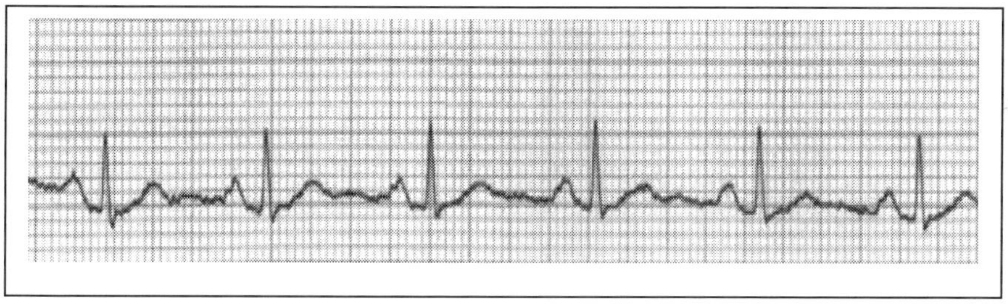

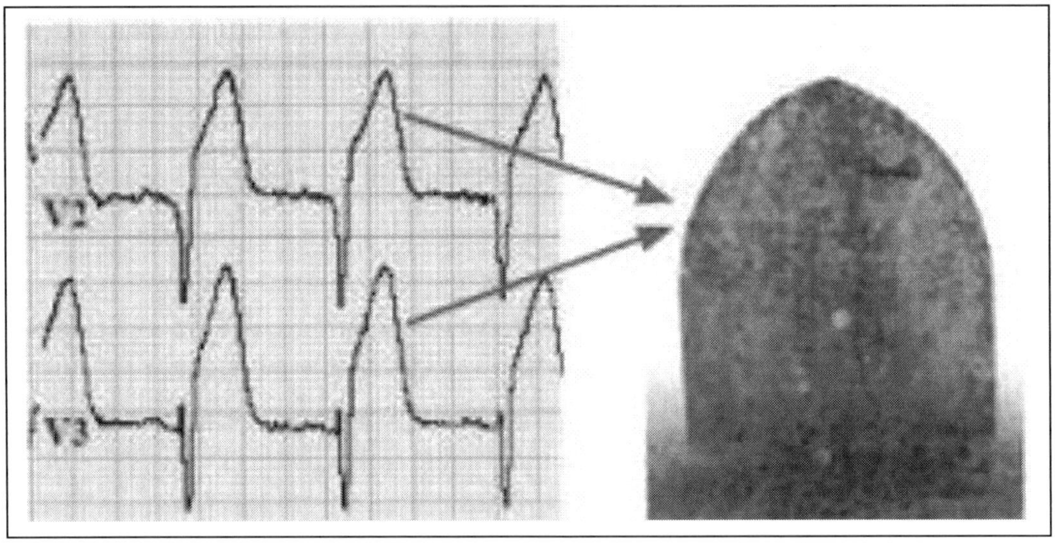

What does an MI look like?

When the discussion of a Myocardial Infarction (MI) turns to reading EKG's there are some things you should look for in the strip. Initially there is an event called a Premature Ventricular Contraction (PVC) that is a marker that should be watched. The PVC is a single focus cell in the ventricles that fire out of turn. Depending on the location the tracing may appear different. If the PVC tracing is the same the beat will be considered Unifocal. If the PVC tracing has different looking beats then it considered to be Multifocal.

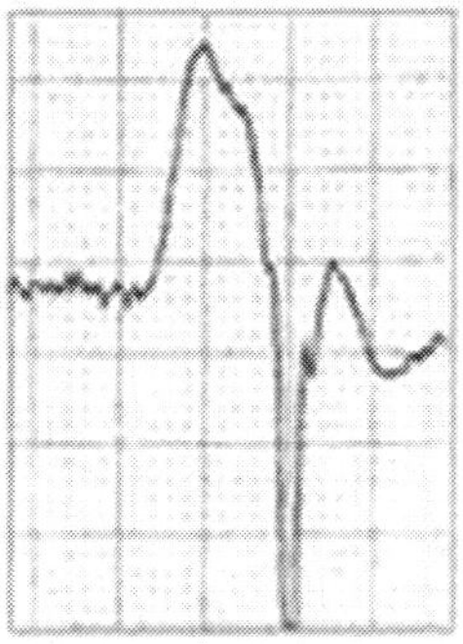

PVC

If the PVC's begin to link together then a rhythm call Bigeminy. In this condition we will see a PVC intermingled evenly with Sinus beats.

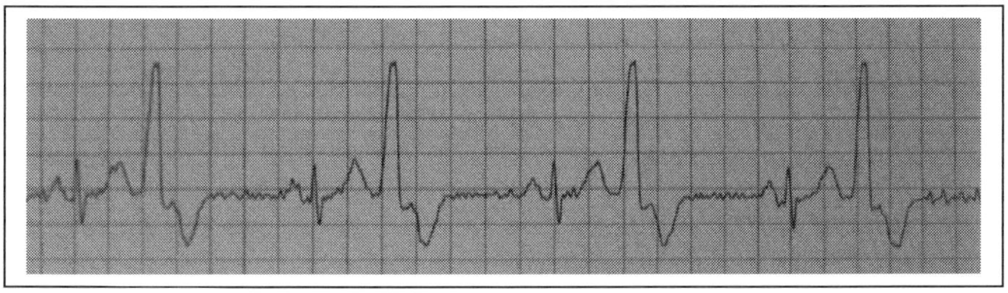

Additionally a condition known as Trigeminy can also be seen where a PVC will fall every 3rd beat.

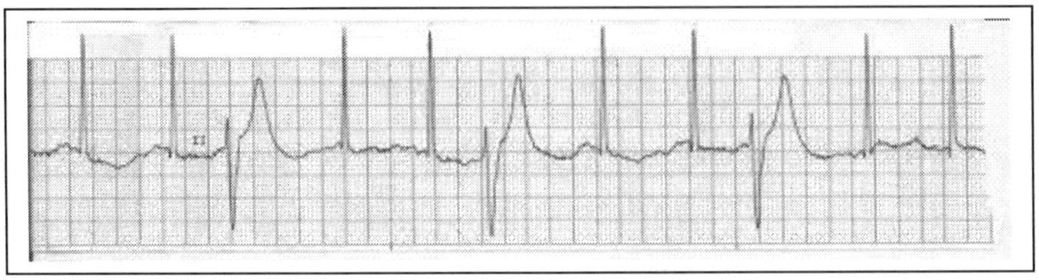

Any time you have PVC's in your patients rhythm you should count them over a minute and report the findings to your medical control. Additionally you may be required by protocol to treat the PVC's before the roll into a more lethal VTach or other associated rhythm. In any circumstance your patient should be treated with care and not bounced around to excessively.

**** A note worth mentioning. Every one of us have a PVC every now and then. However it becomes significant when the number of PVC's reach six or more a minute, especially if the patient has had no surgical event in their history.

"T" waves are the next segment of the complex which should be looked at very contentiously. The "T" wave is an indicator of how the heart is receiving Oxygenated blood. If the "T" wave begins to flatten it may be significant to electrolyte disturbances such as dehydration. However, if the "T" wave inverts or is in opposite direction of the "QRS" complex then ischemia (lack of oxygen) has or is occurring in the heart. These patients should be interviewed well and your best efforts should be made to determine the etiology of the change in the "T" waves.

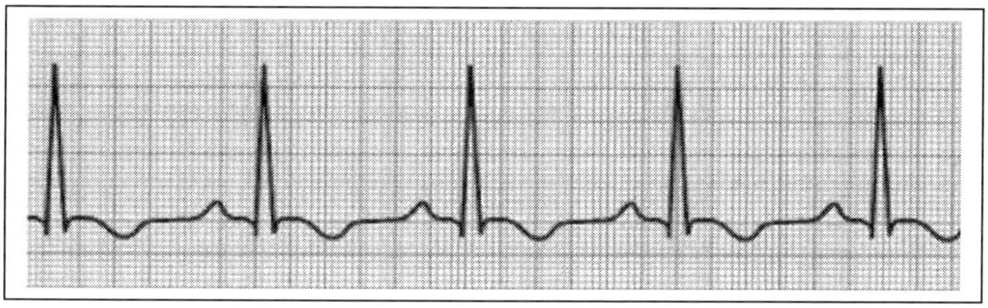

When the "T" wave has left the base line the patient is either entering into a Myocardial Infarction (MI) or coming out of one. Definitive laboratory results will identify the place on the time line for the doctor. That being said, for our purposes, unless you are in a place where there is active laboratory support consider all patients in this position to be entering into a Cardiac event and treat per your protocol and ACLS directives. These patients can be fragile and can make a turn for the worse with little or no warning. Be prepared for the worst.

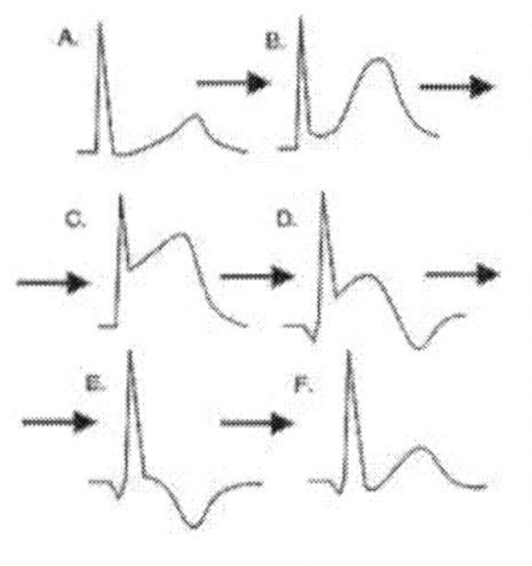

MI Progression

"Q" waves are the next and most misdiagnosed Marker you should consider. The "Q" wave to be Considered significant must be at least 2/3's the size of the "RS" wave complex. Many patients have been brought to emergency rooms with the diagnosis of "MI with Q waves present". The misdiagnosis in this situation is OK; the reason being the patient will be treated per protocol for an active MI and nothing will be missed. When it is all said and done the Doctor in the Emergency Room is the one to make the call. The Doctor wont usually make the diagnosis on the presence of a "Q" wave in an EKG alone. Definitive labs and a intact symptomology is also important.

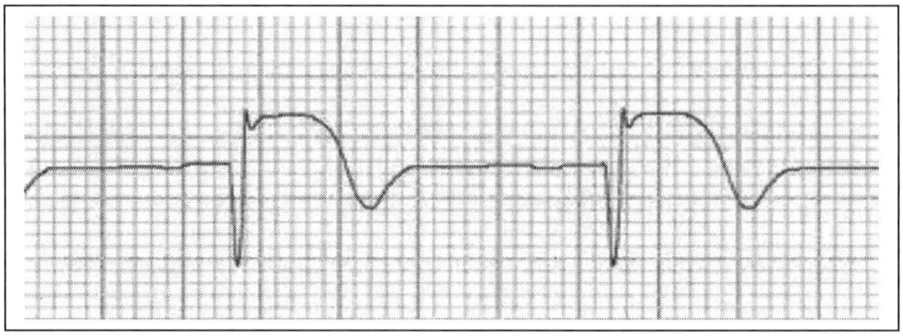

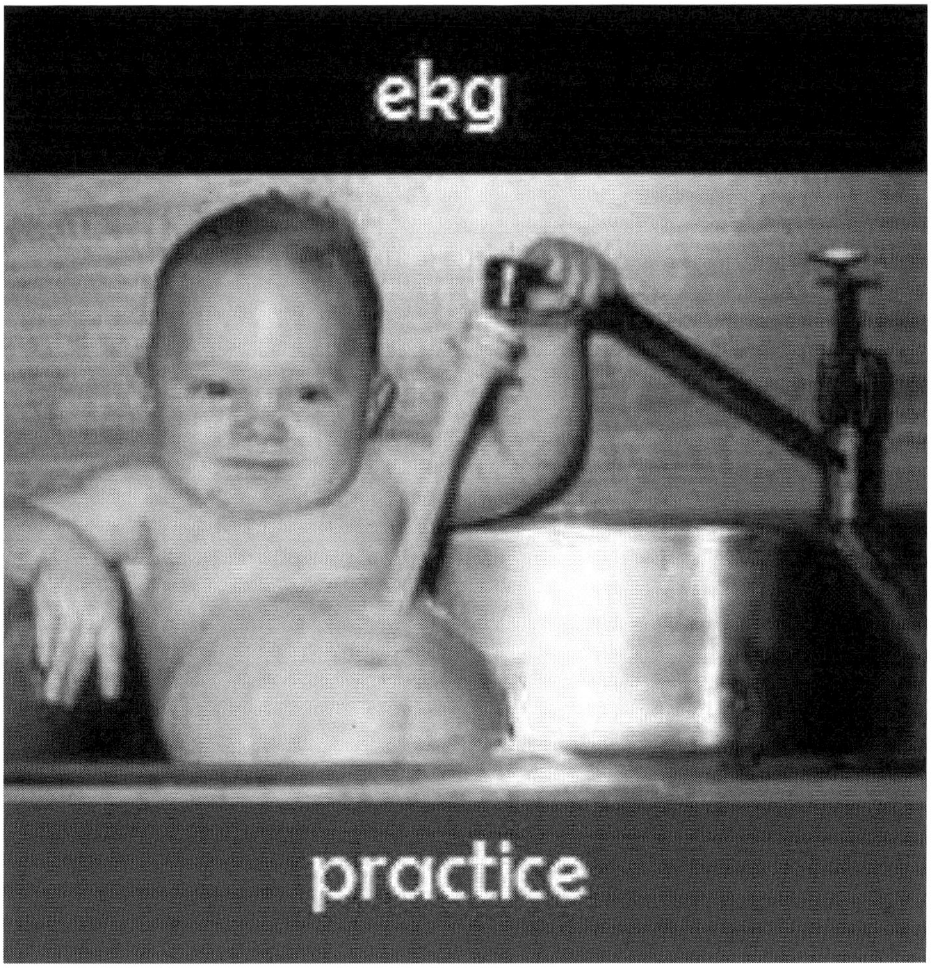

Let's put it all together an go over a few. Each strip is numbered and the interpretation is in the back of the book. Take your time and use tour rules we have discussed to work through each strip. If you get stuck it is OK, try to determine if the rhythm originated in the atrium or the ventricles then start applying the accordingly.

- Medicsmith

1

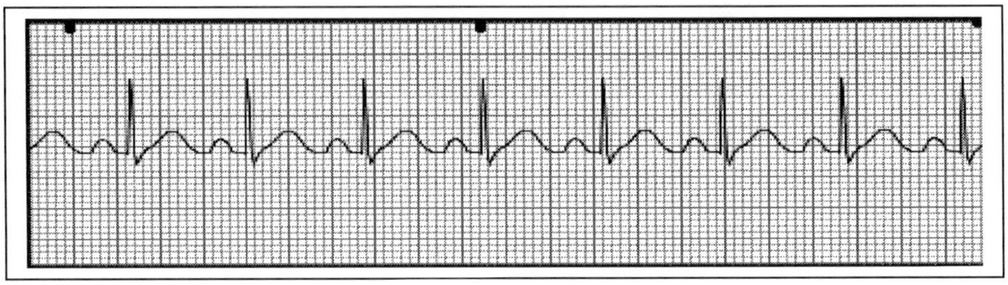

Interpretation: ____

Rate: _____________

2

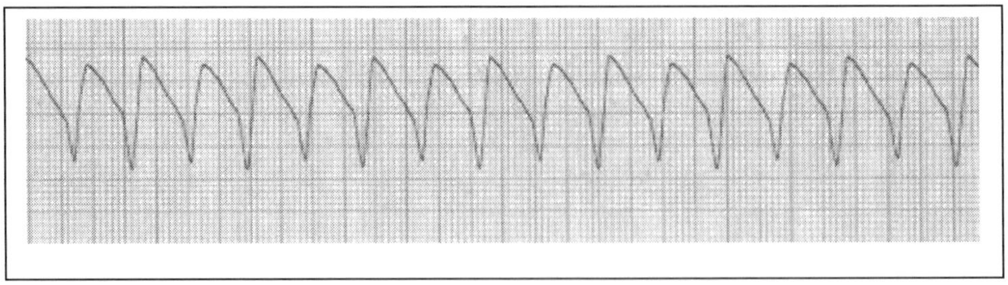

Interpretation: ____

Rate: ______________

3

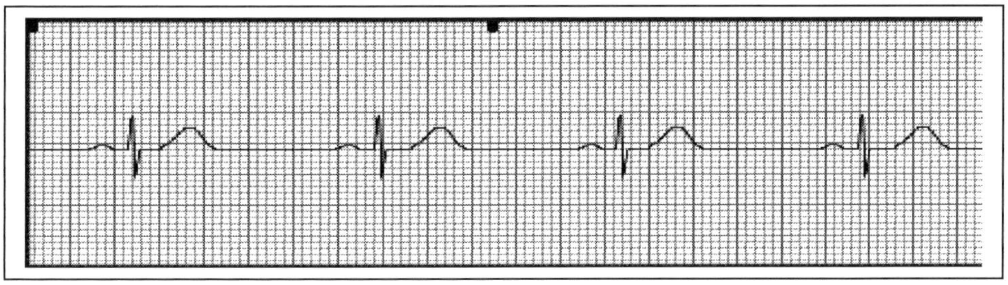

Interpretation: ______________________________

Rate: __________

4

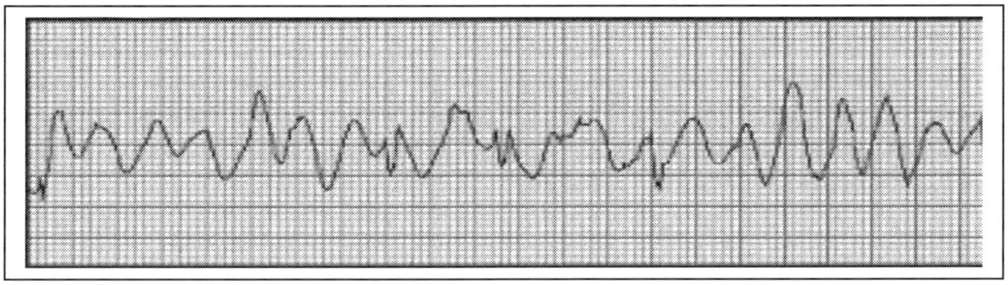

Interpretation: ______________________________

Rate: __________

5

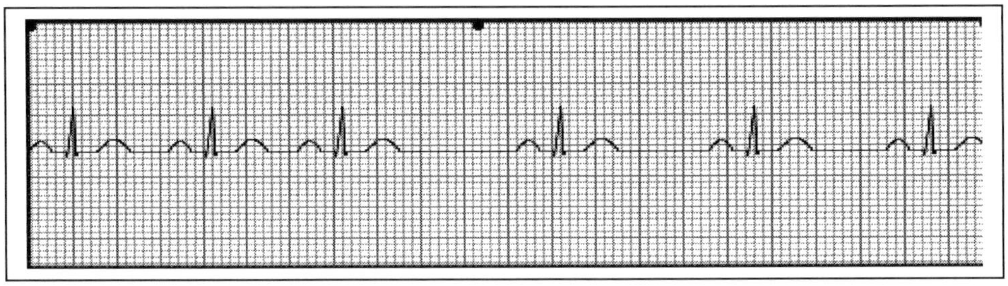

Interpretation: ______________________________

Rate: __________

6

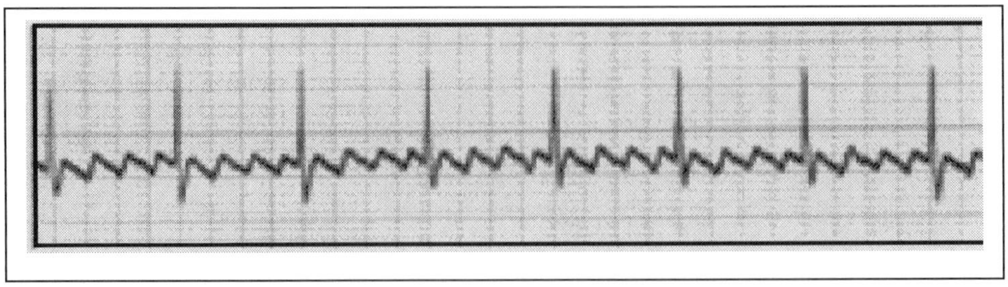

Interpretation: ______________________________

Rate: __________

7

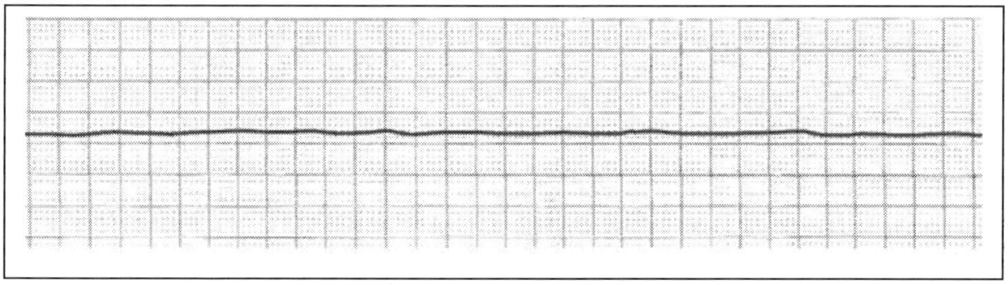

Interpretation: ________________________________

Rate: ___________

8

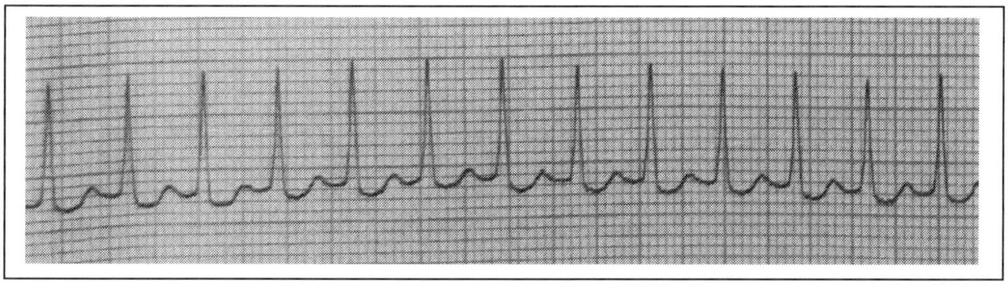

Interpretation: ________________________________

Rate: ____________

9

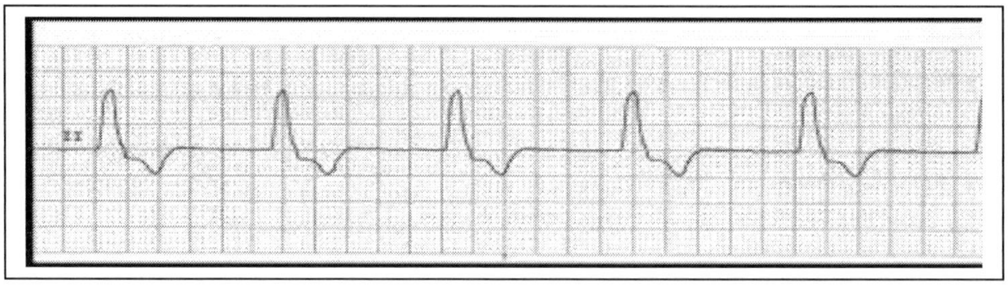

Interpretation: ____________________________________

Rate: ____________

10

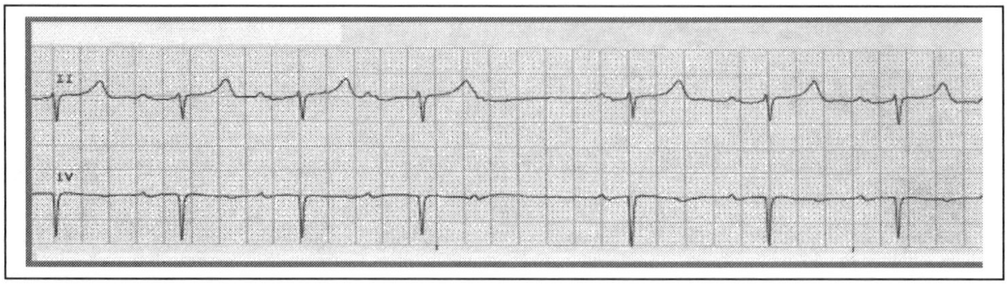

Interpretation: ____________________________________

Rate: _____________

11

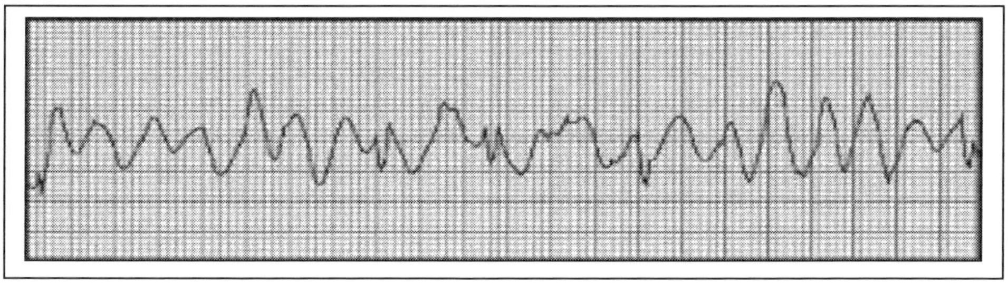

Interpretation: ___________________________________

Rate: ____________

12

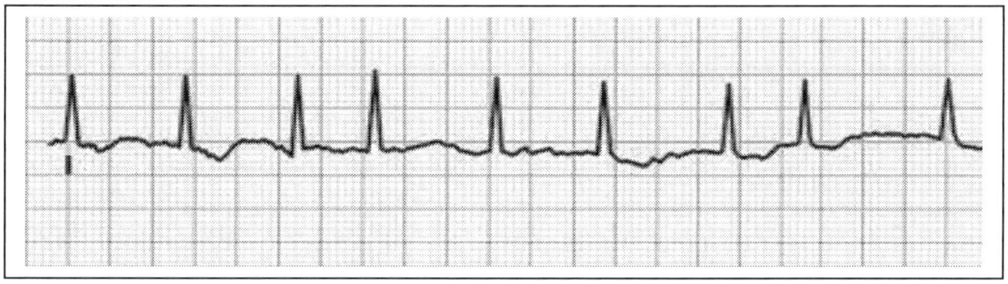

Interpretation: ___________________________________

Rate: _____________

13

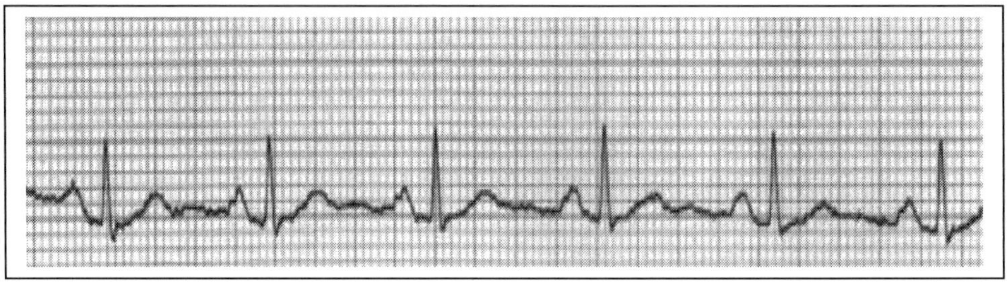

Interpretation: ___________________________________

Rate: ___________

14

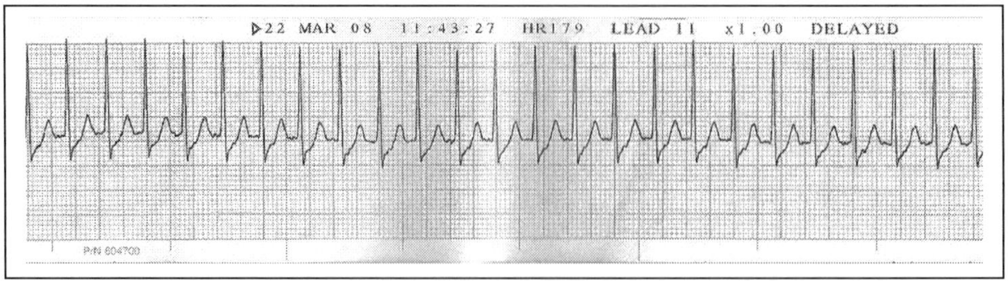

Interpretation: ___________________________________

Rate: ____________

15

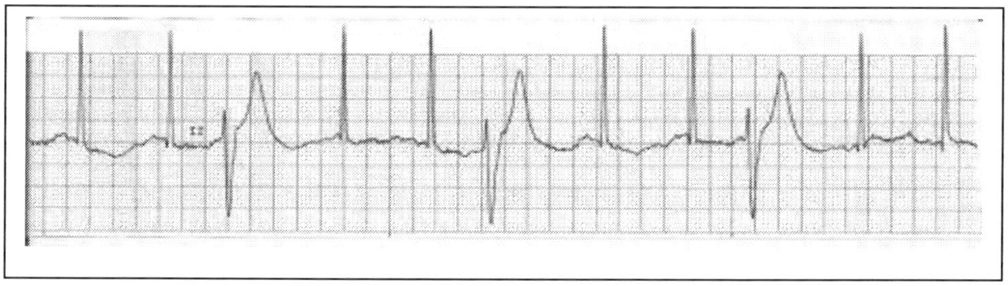

Interpretation: ____________________________________

Rate: ____________

16

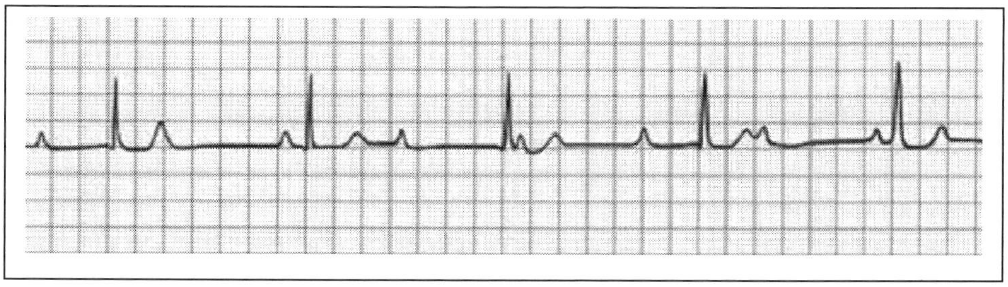

Interpretation: ____________________________________

Rate: _____________

17

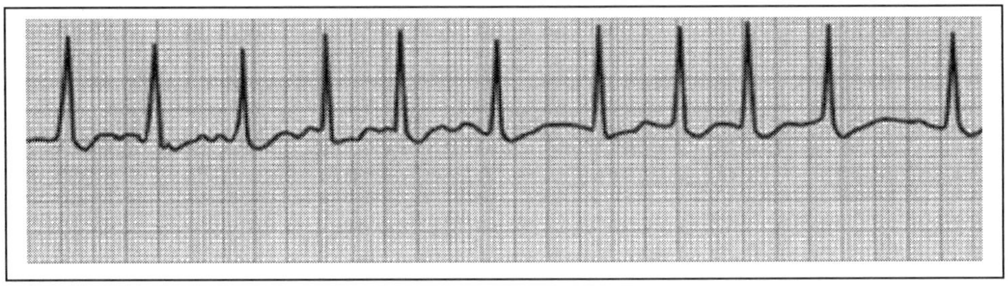

Interpretation: ________________________________

Rate: ____________

18

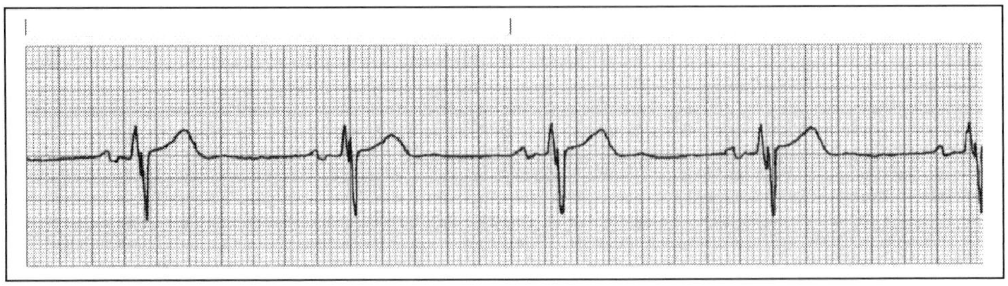

Interpretation: ________________________________

Rate: ____________

19

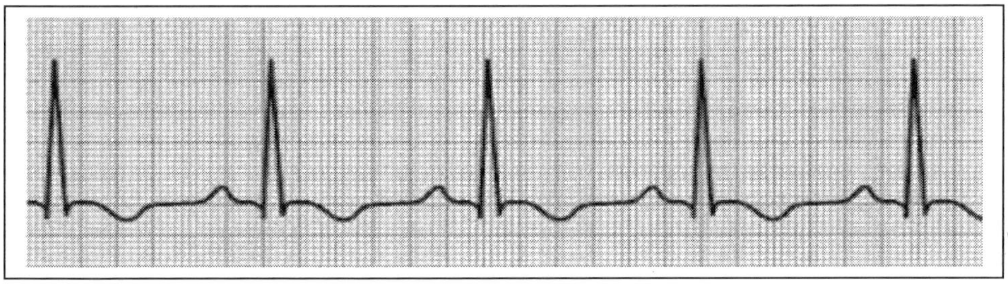

Interpretation: ______________________________

Rate: __________

20

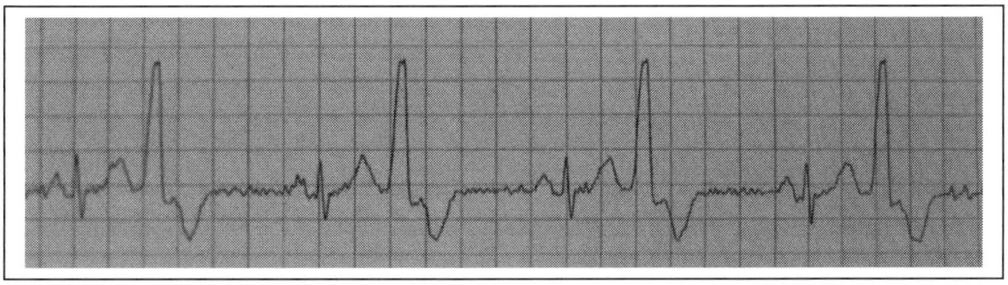

Interpretation: ______________________________

Rate: ___________

21

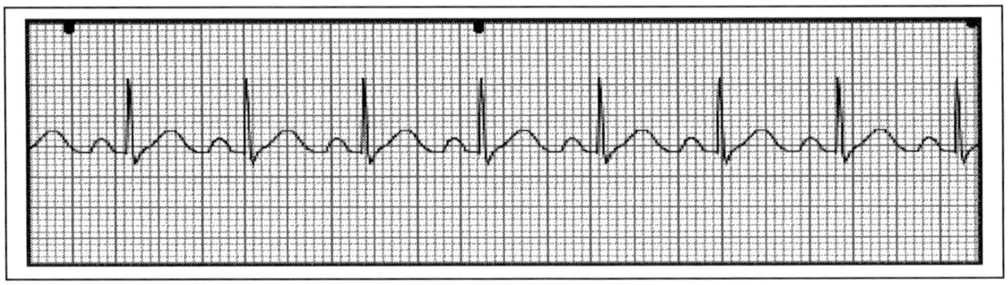

Interpretation: ______________________________

Rate: __________

22

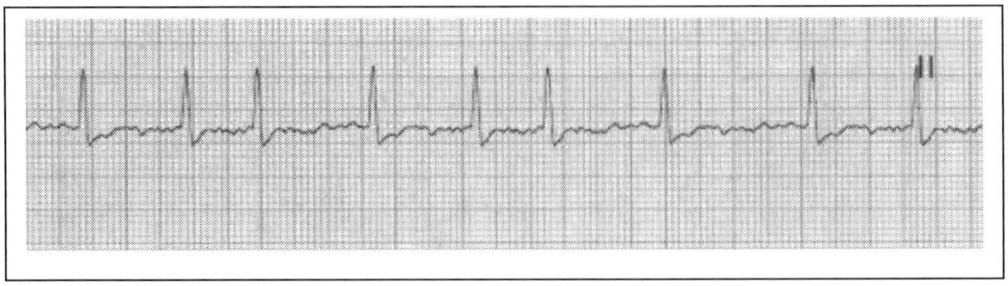

Interpretation: ______________________________

Rate: __________

23

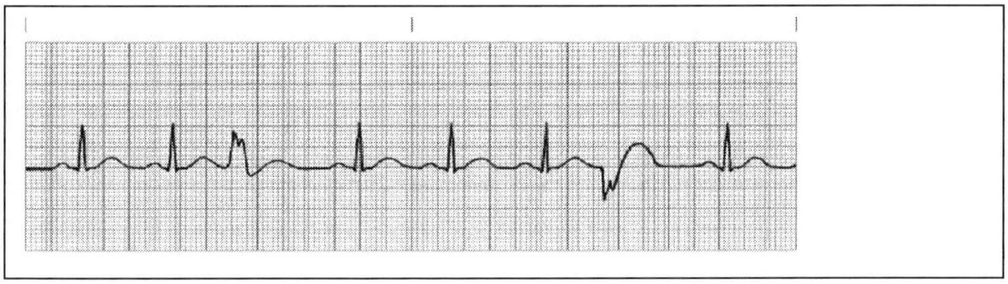

Interpretation: ________________________________

Rate: ___________

24

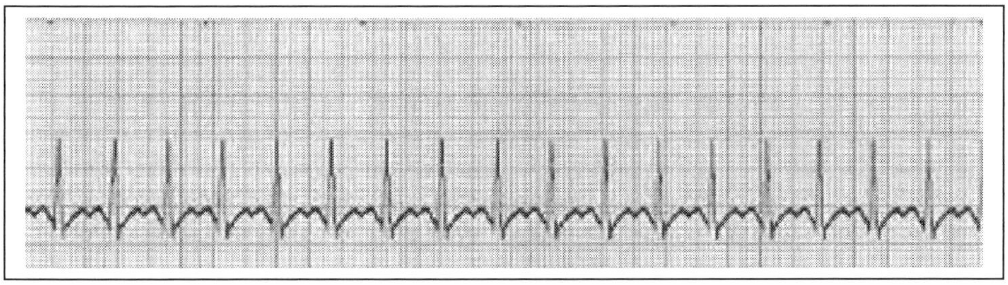

Interpretation: ________________________________

Rate: ____________

25

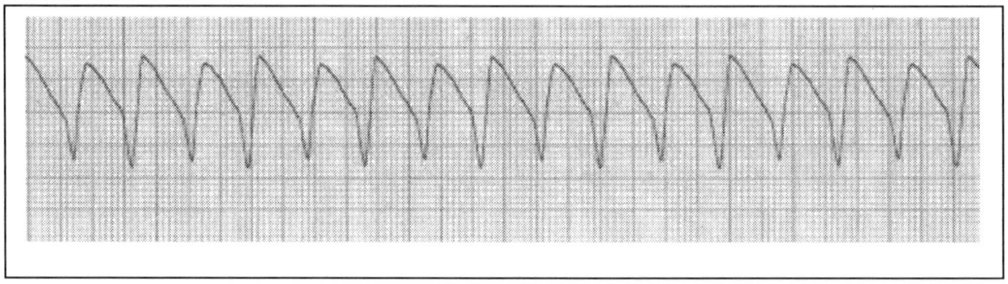

Interpretation: ______________________________

Rate: __________

26

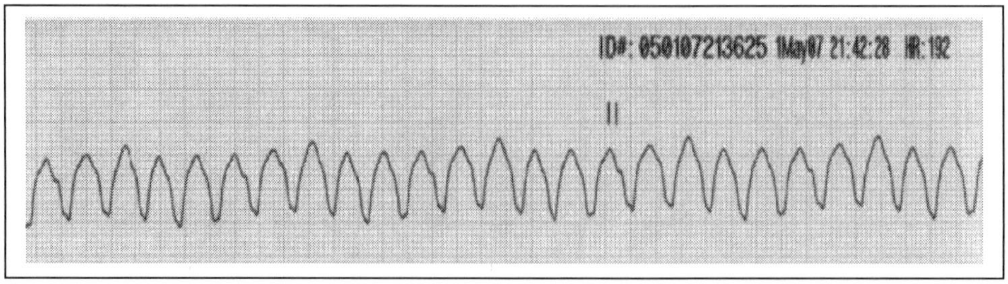

Interpretation: ______________________________

Rate: __________

27

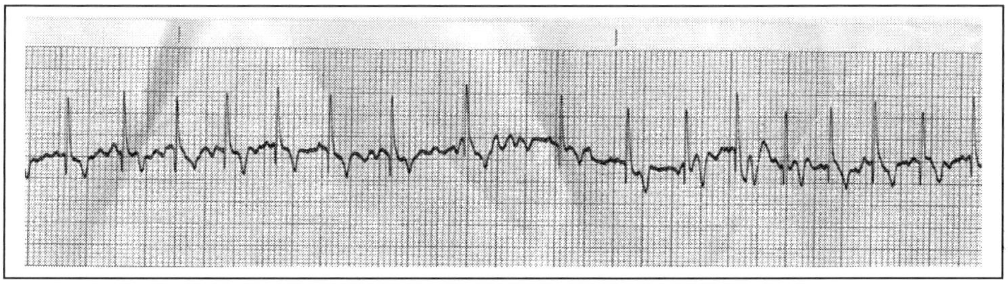

Interpretation: ___________________________________

Rate: ____________

28

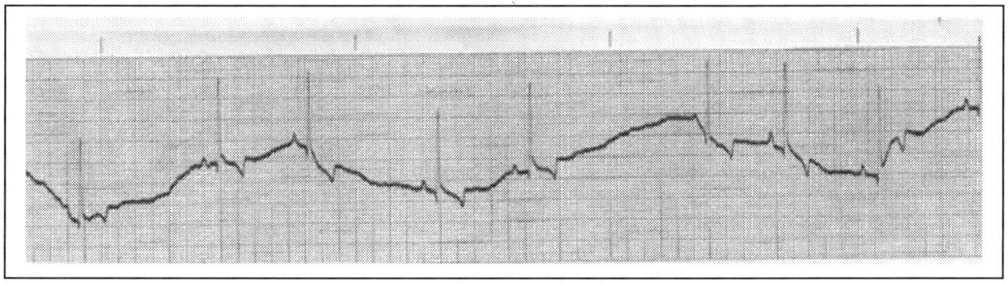

Interpretation: ___________________________________

Rate: _____________

29

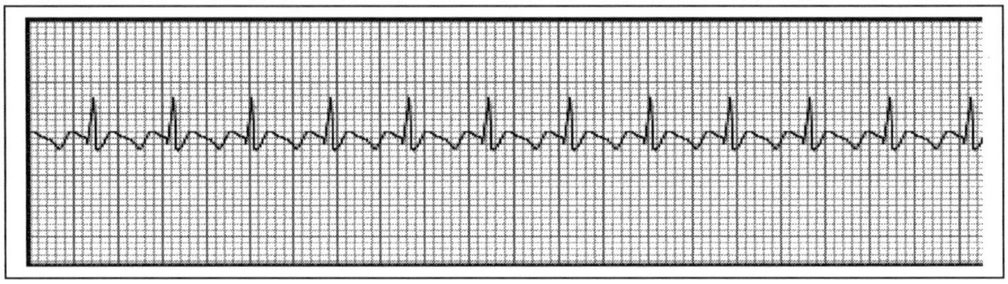

Interpretation: ________________________________

Rate: __________

30

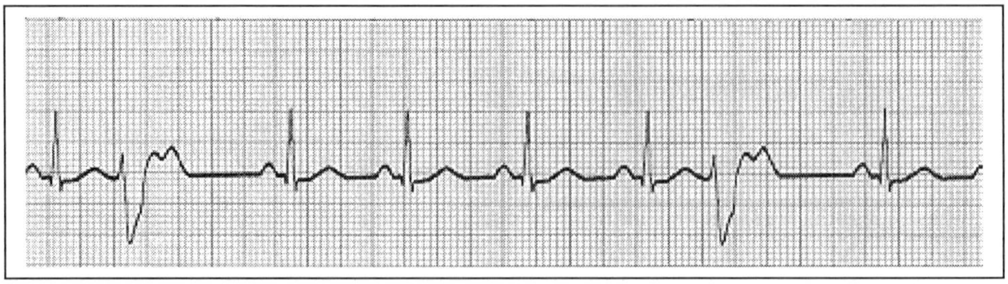

Interpretation: ________________________________

Rate: __________

31

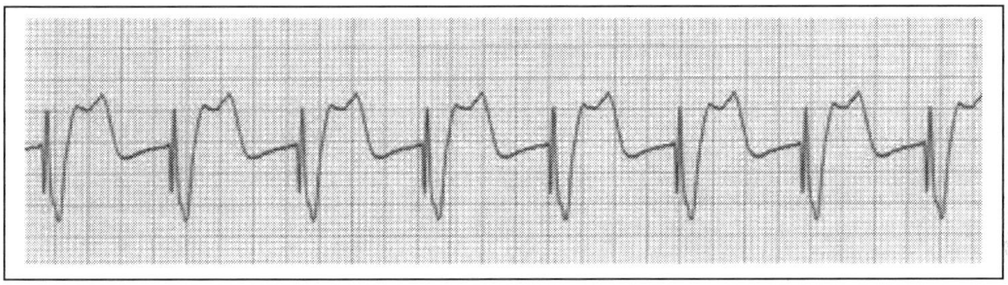

Interpretation: ___________________________________

Rate: ____________

32

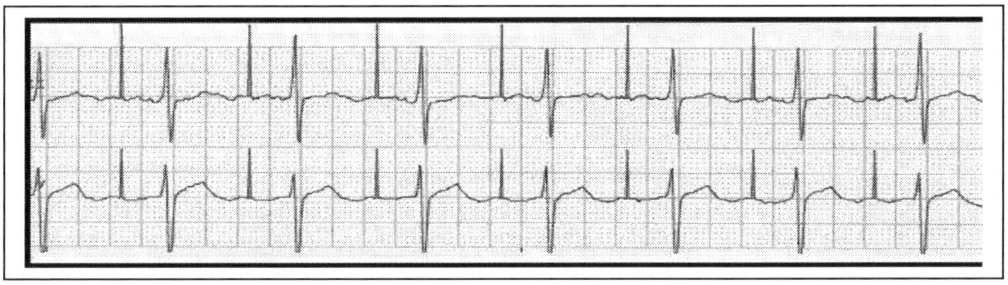

Interpretation: ___________________________________

Rate: _____________

33

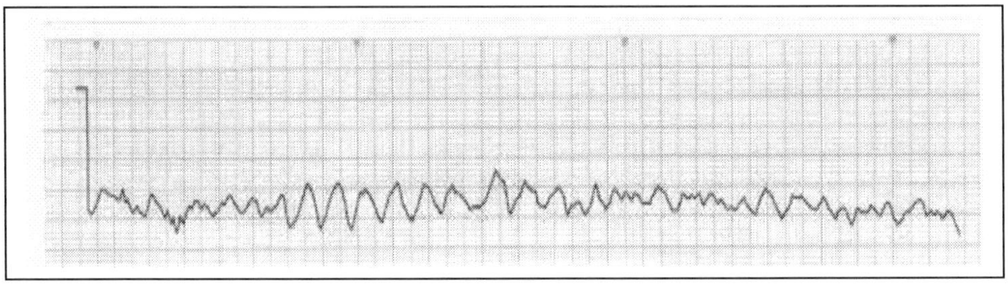

Interpretation: ________________________________

Rate: __________

34

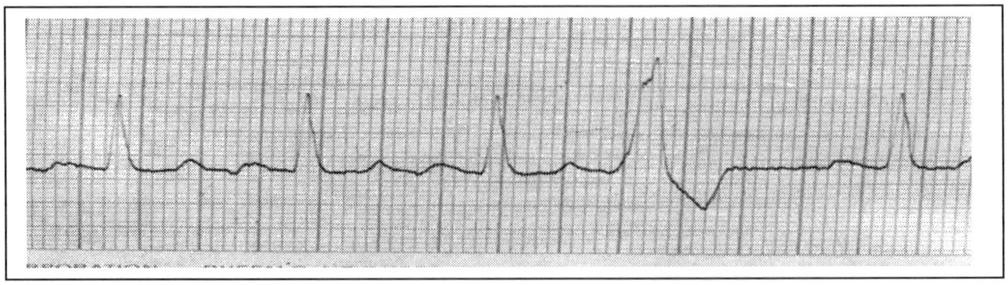

Interpretation: ________________________________

Rate: __________

35

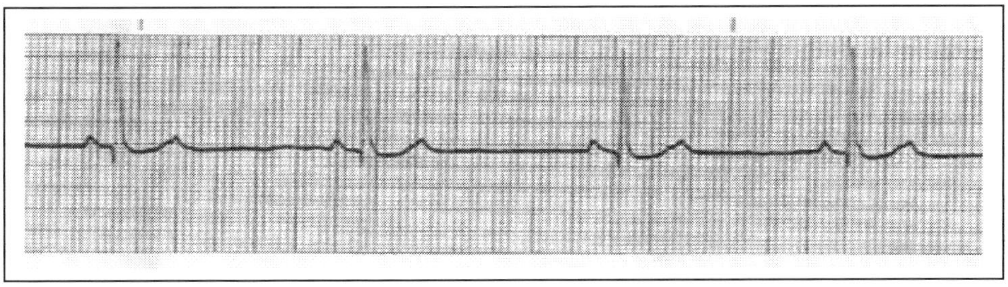

Interpretation: ______________________________

Rate: __________

36

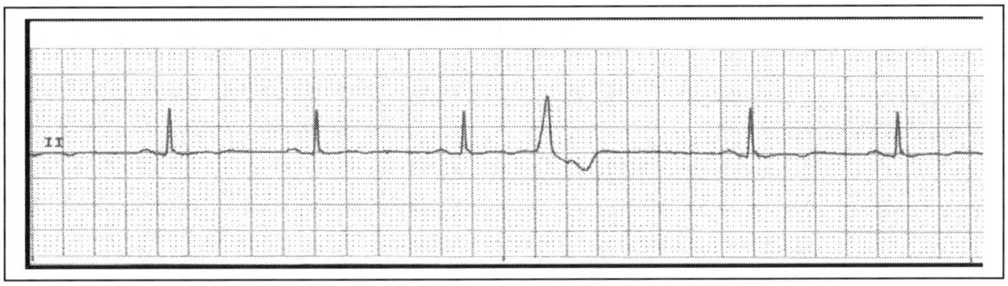

Interpretation: ______________________________

Rate: __________

37

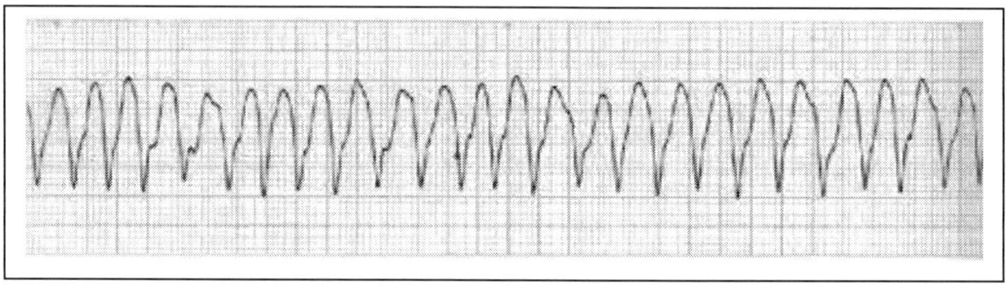

Interpretation: ________________________________

Rate: ___________

38

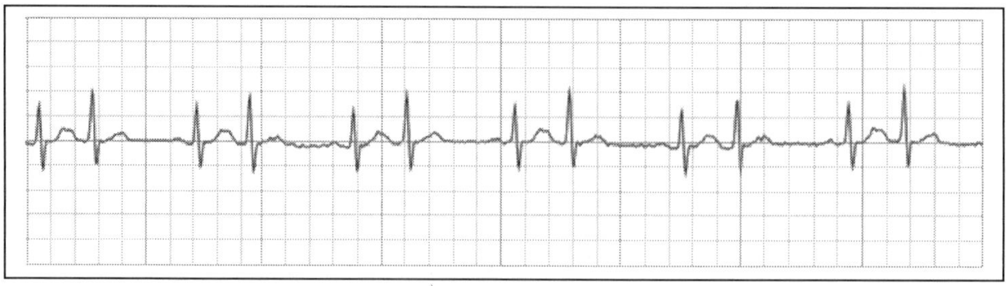

Interpretation: ________________________________

Rate: ___________

39

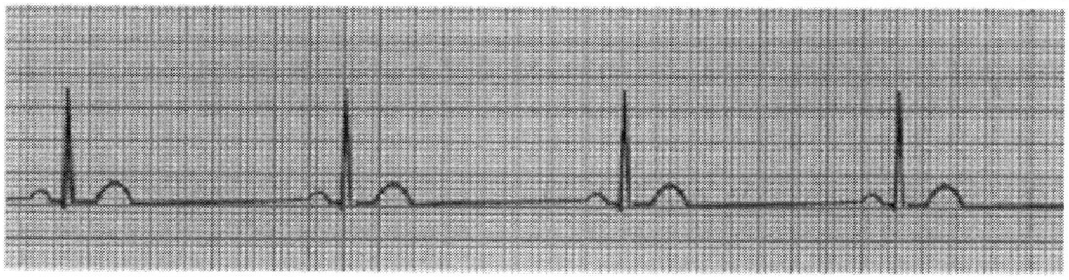

Interpretation: ______________________________

Rate: __________

40

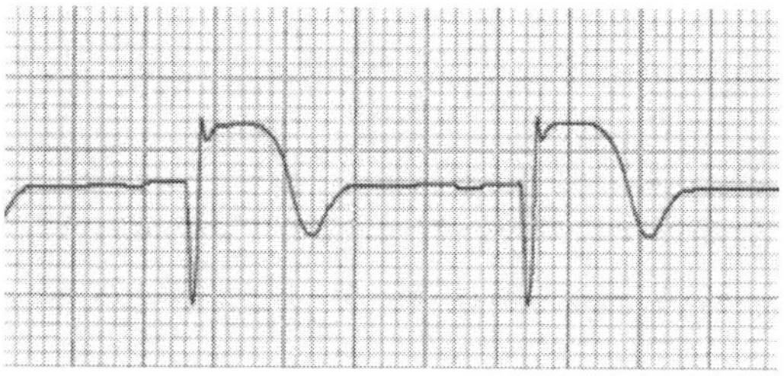

Interpretation: ______________________________

Rate: __________

41

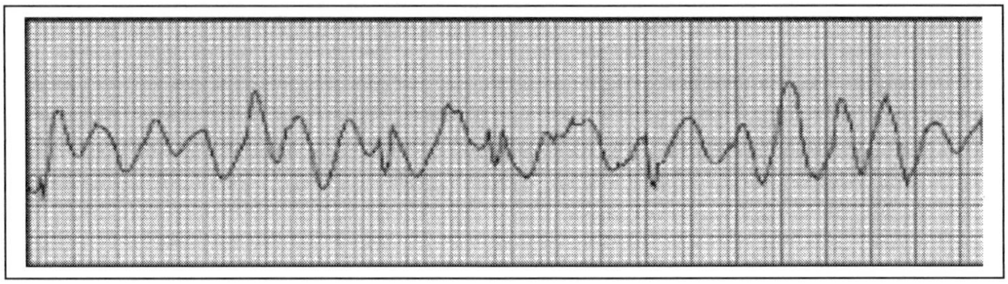

Interpretation: ___________________________________

Rate: ___________

42

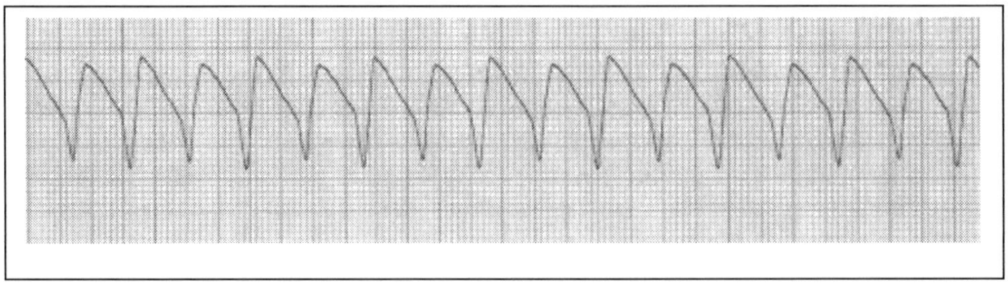

Interpretation: ___________________________________

Rate: ____________

43

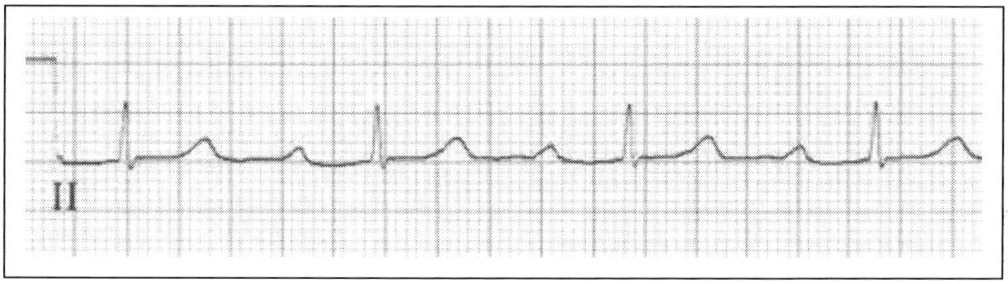

Interpretation: ______________________________

Rate: __________

44

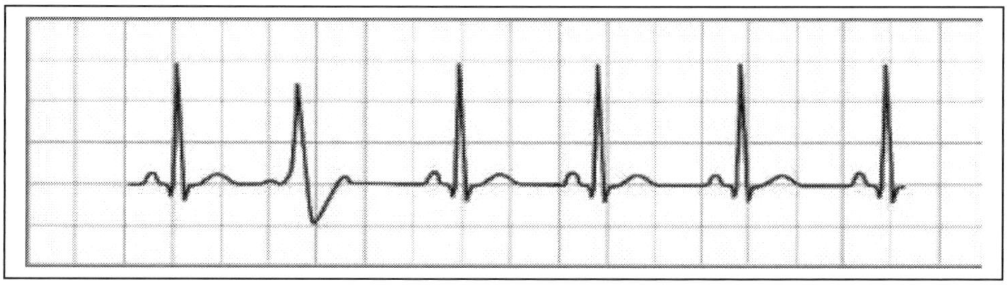

Interpretation: ______________________________

Rate: ___________

45

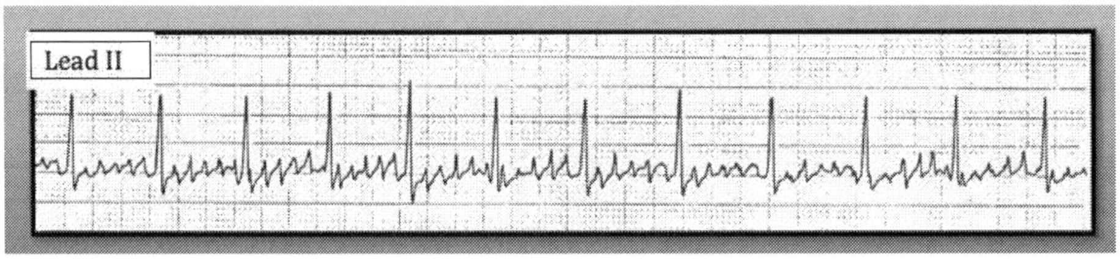

Interpretation: ________________________________

Rate: ___________

46

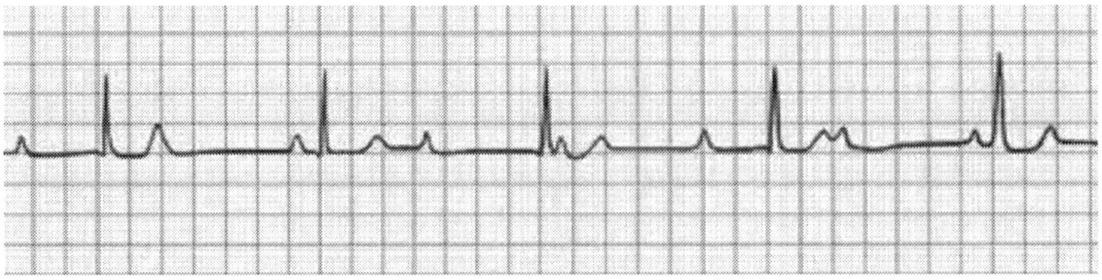

Interpretation: ________________________________

Rate: ___________

47

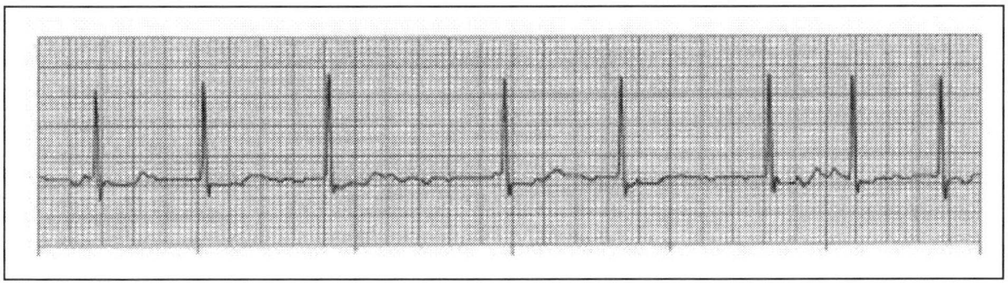

Interpretation: ____________________________________

Rate: ____________

48

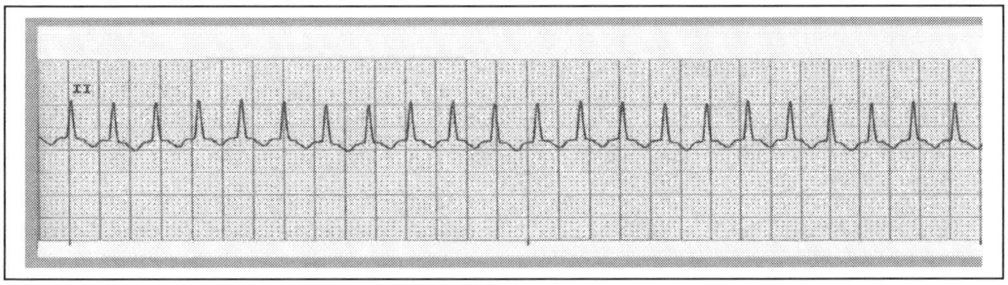

Interpretation: ____________________________________

Rate: _____________

49

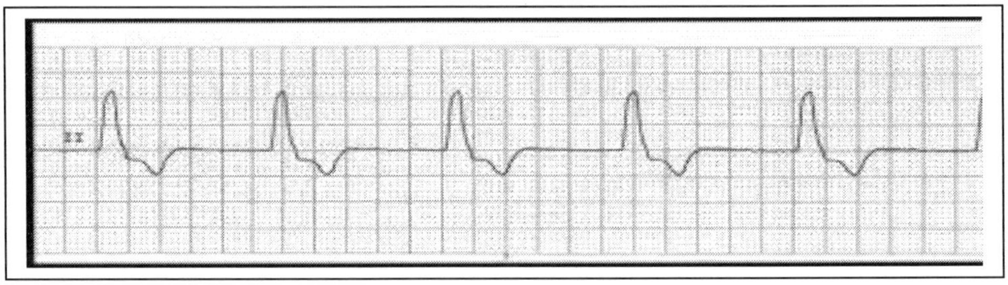

Interpretation: ________________________________

Rate: ___________

50

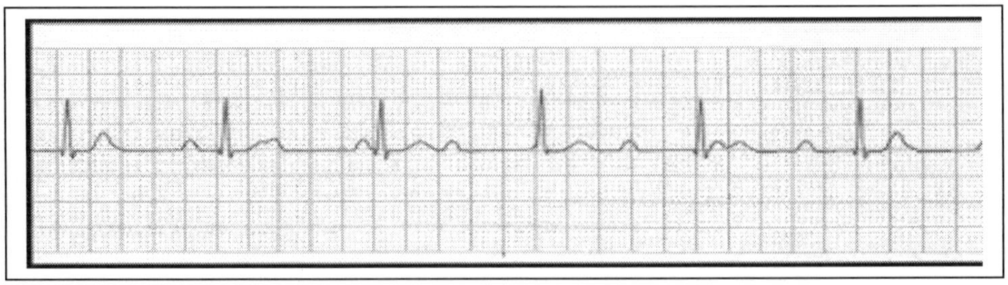

Interpretation: ________________________________

Rate: ___________

51

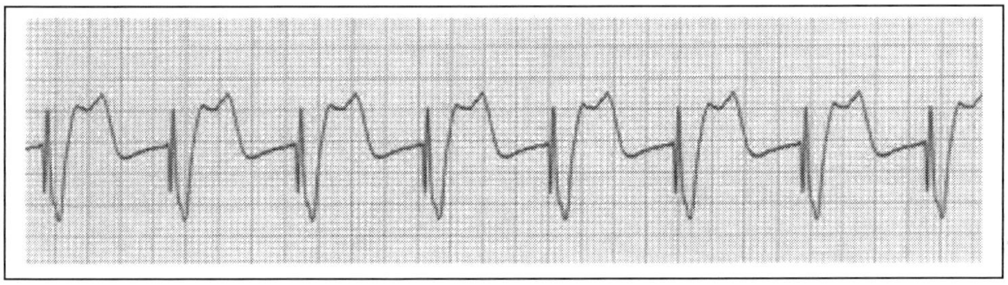

Interpretation: ___________________________________

Rate: ___________

52

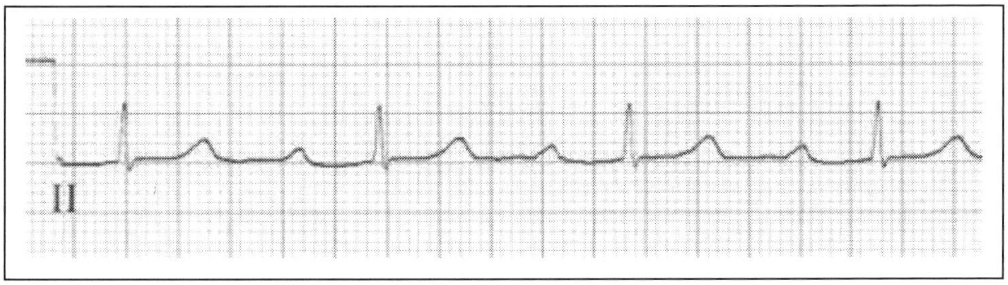

Interpretation: ___________________________________

Rate: ____________

53

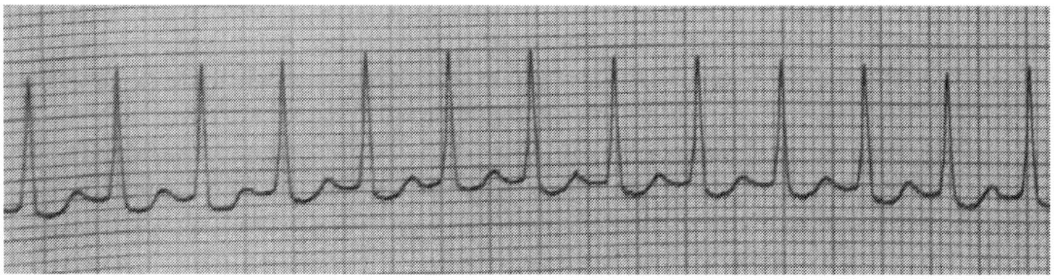

Interpretation: ________________________________

Rate: ___________

54

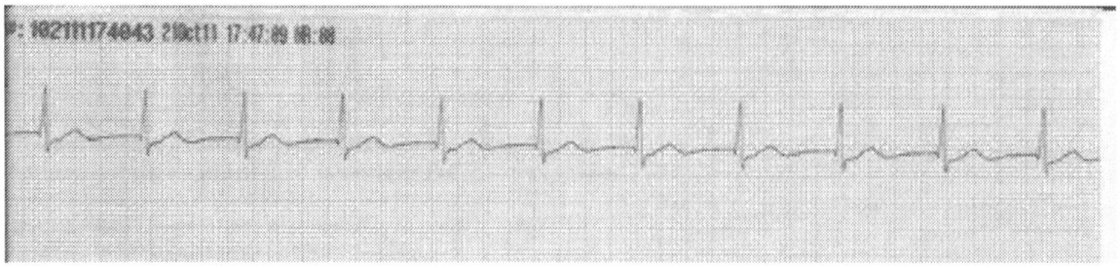

Interpretation: ________________________________

Rate: ___________

55

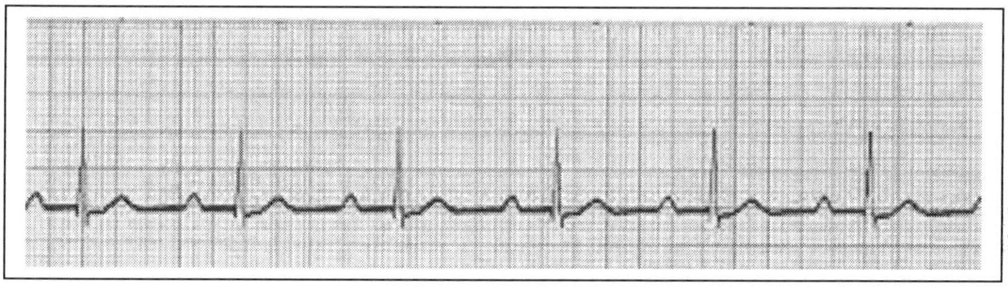

Interpretation: ______________________________

Rate: __________

56

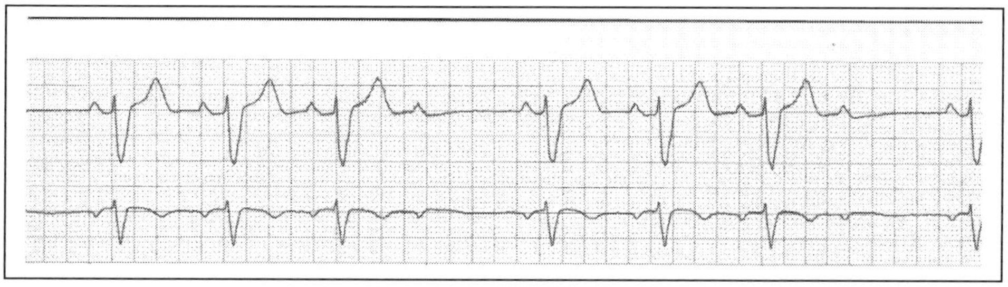

Interpretation: ______________________________

Rate: __________

57

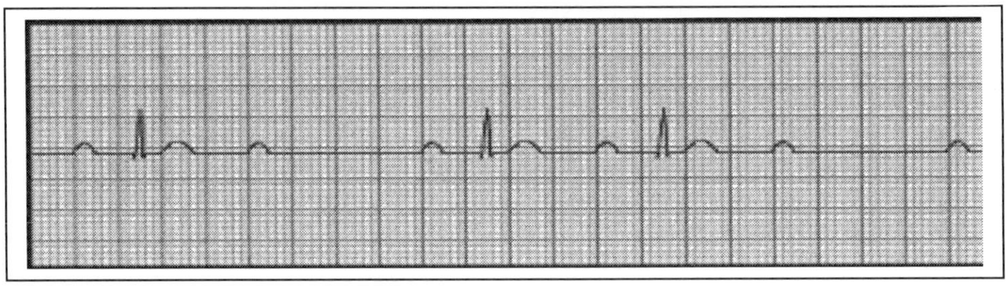

Interpretation: ______________________________

Rate: __________

58

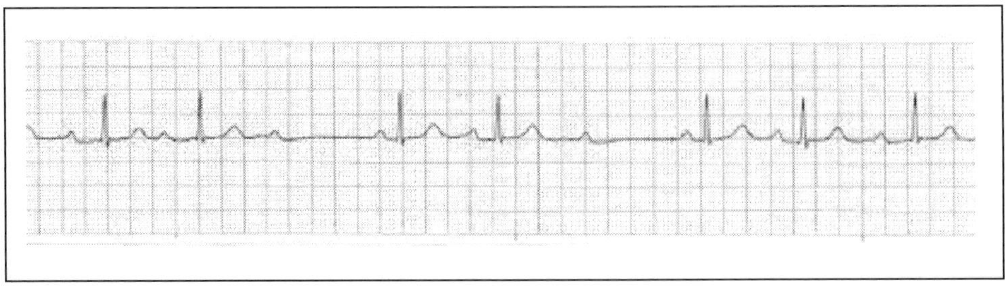

Interpretation: ______________________________

Rate: __________

59

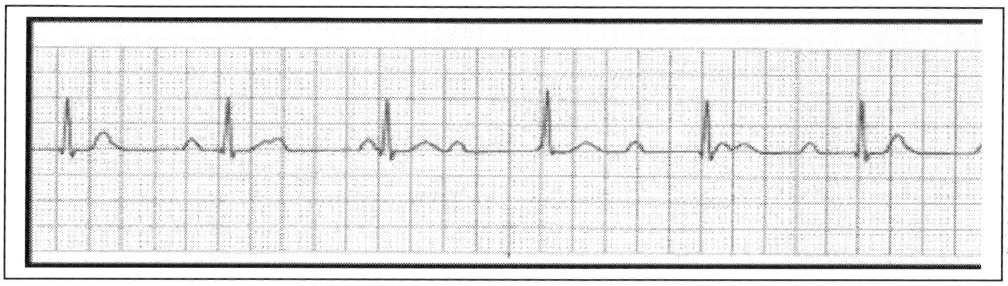

Interpretation: ______________________________

Rate: __________

60

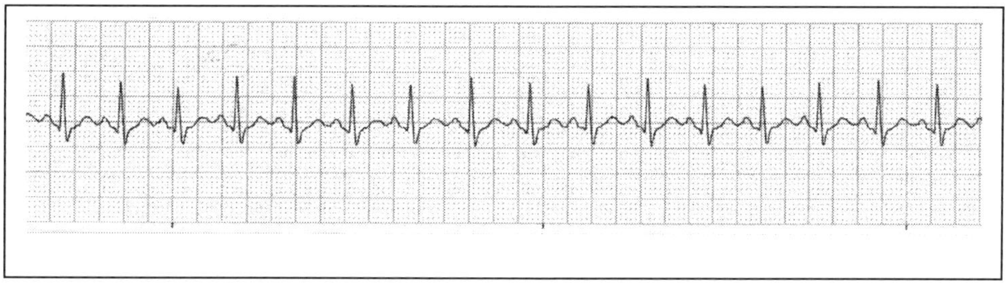

Interpretation: ______________________________

Rate: __________

61

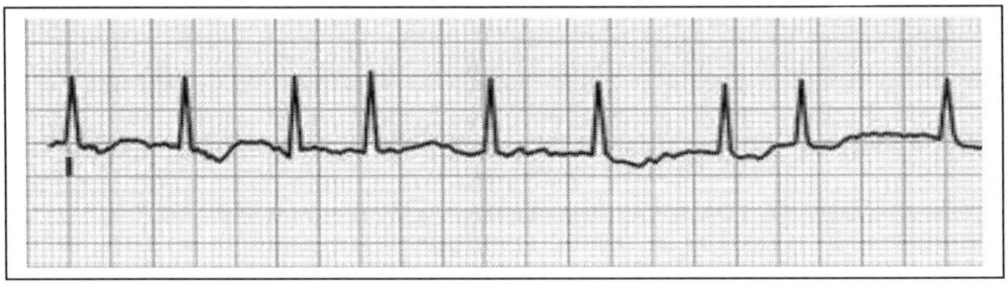

Interpretation: ________________________________

Rate: __________

62

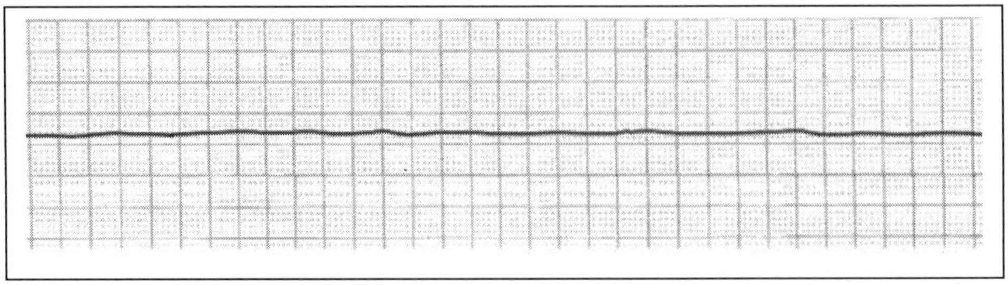

Interpretation: ________________________________

Rate: __________

63

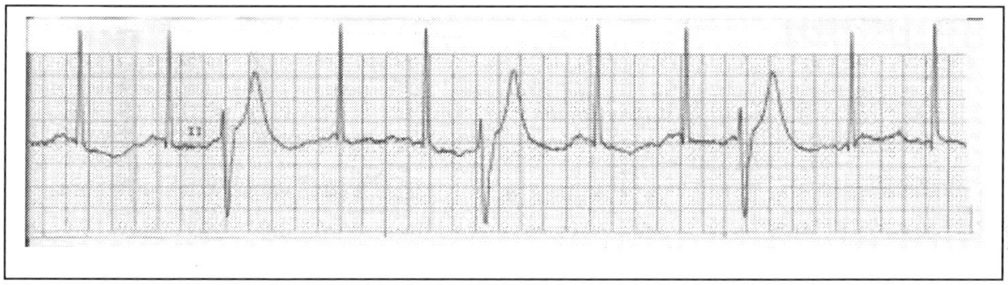

Interpretation: ______________________________

Rate: ____________

64

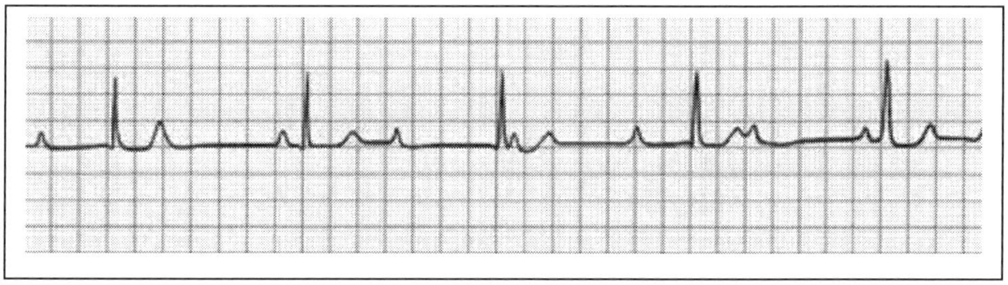

Interpretation: ______________________________

Rate: ____________

65

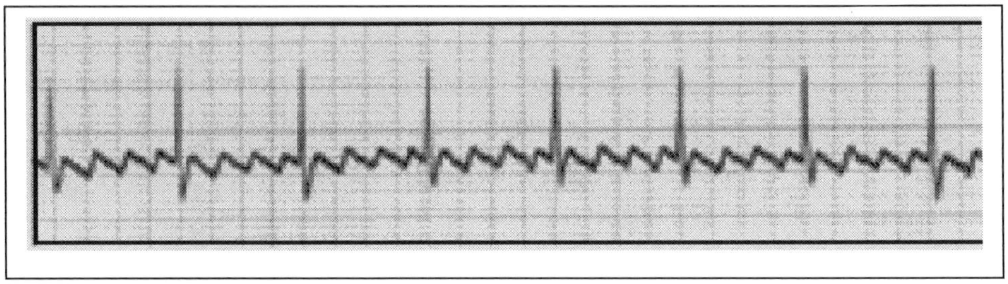

Interpretation: ______________________________________

Rate: ____________

66

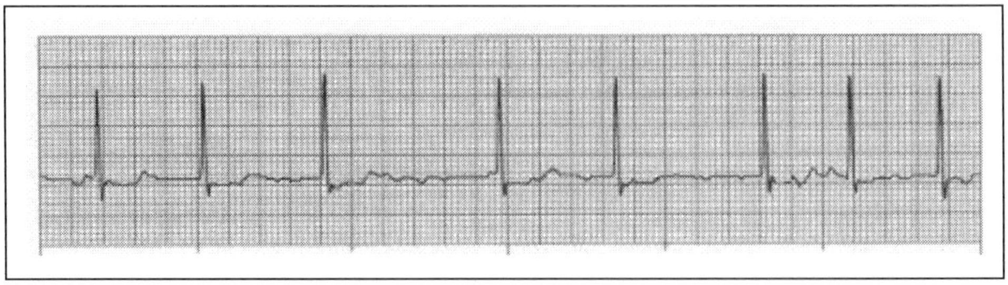

Interpretation: ______________________________________

Rate: _____________

67

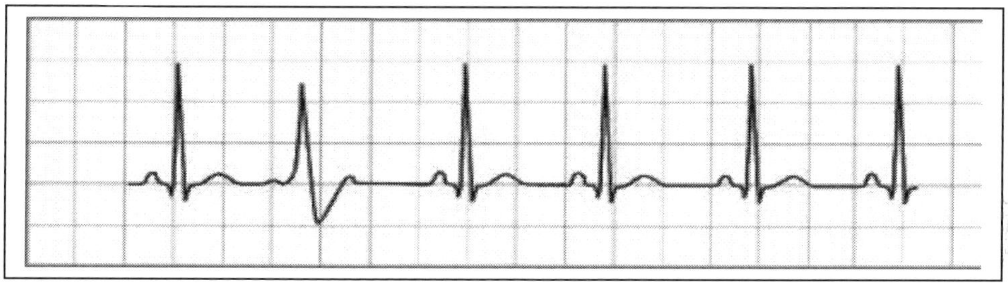

Interpretation: ______________________________

Rate: __________

68

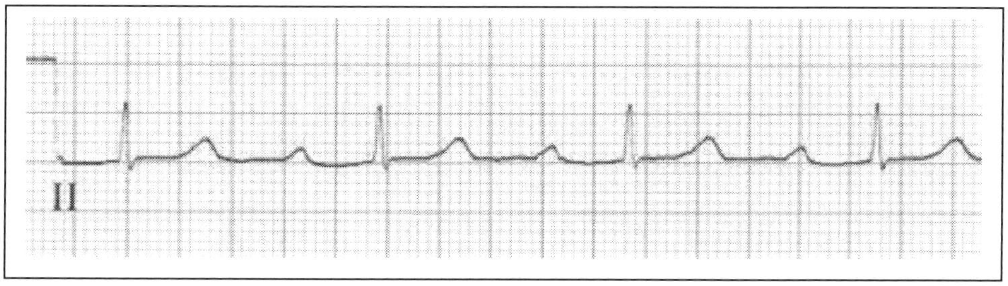

Interpretation: ______________________________

Rate: __________

69

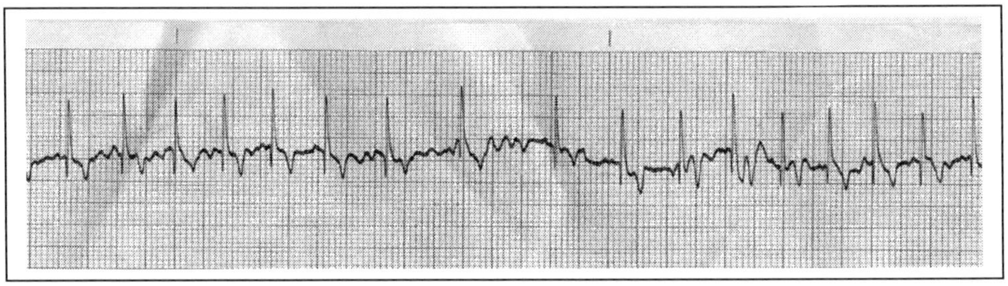

Interpretation: ________________________________

Rate: ___________

70

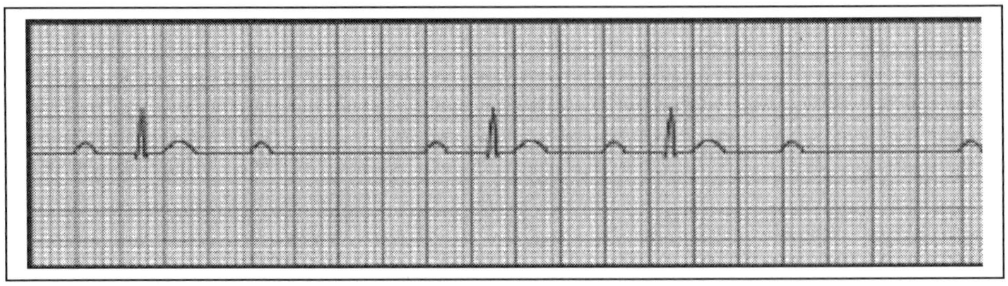

Interpretation: ________________________________

Rate: ___________

71

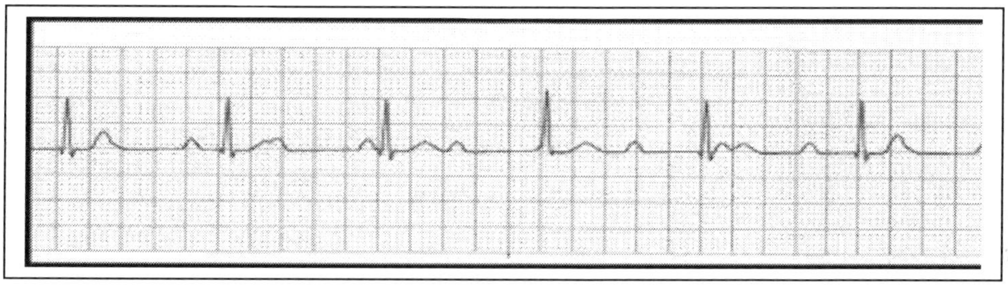

Interpretation: ______________________________

Rate: __________

72

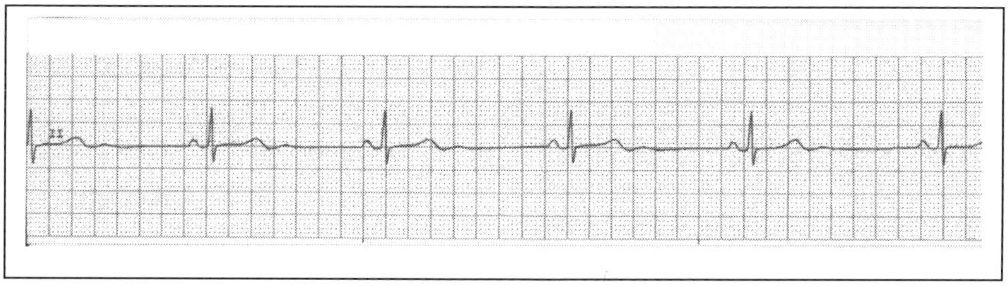

Interpretation: ______________________________

Rate: __________

73

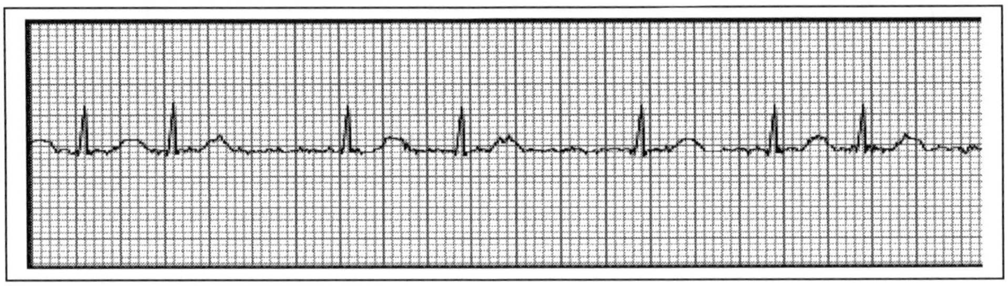

Interpretation: ____________________________________

Rate: ____________

74

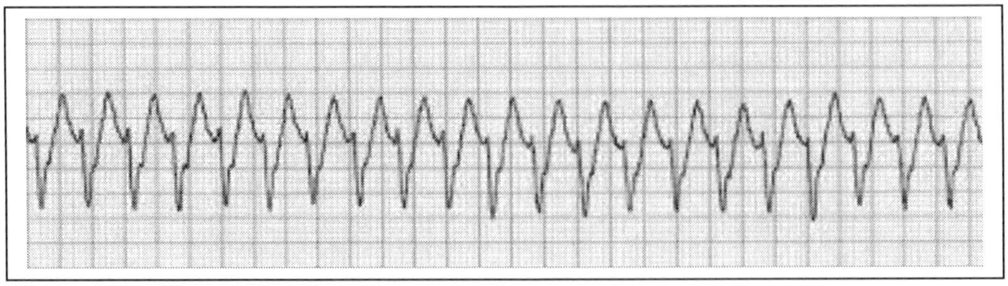

Interpretation: ____________________________________

Rate: _____________

75

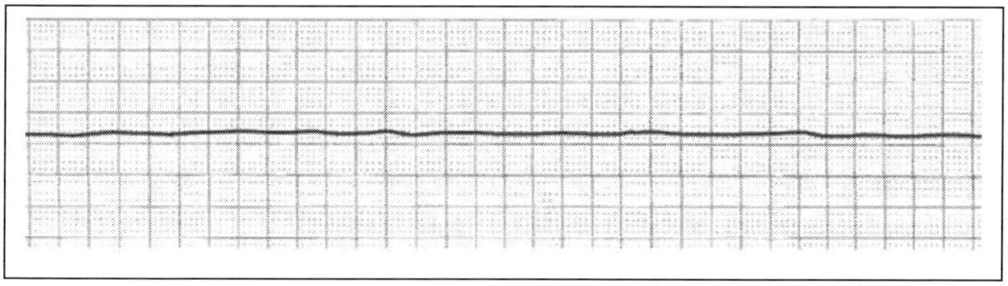

Interpretation: ______________________________

Rate: __________

76

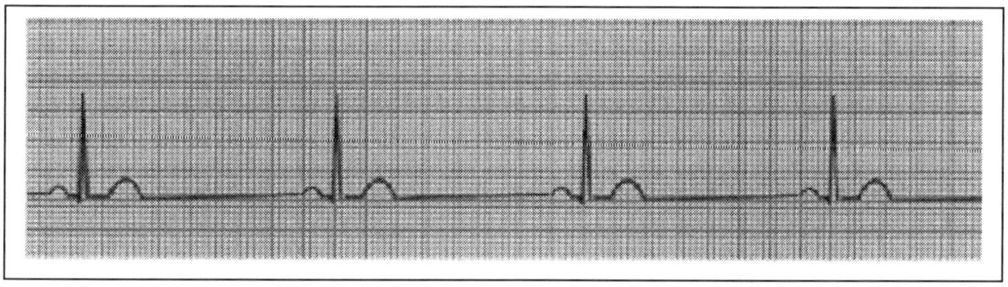

Interpretation: ______________________________

Rate: __________

Interpretation Key

1. NSR
2. VTACH
3. BRADY
4. VFIB
5. SINUS ARREST BEAT
6. AFLUTTER
7. ASYSTOLE
8. ACCELERATED JUNCTIONAL
9. IDIOVENTRICULAR
10. 2ND DEGREE TYPE I
11. VFIB
12. AFIB
13. PEA
14. SVT
15. TRIGEMINY
16. 3RD DEGREE

17.AFLUTTER

18.SINUS BRADY

19.SINUS WITH INVERTED "T" WAVES

20.BIGEMINY

21.NSR

22.AFIB

23.MULTIFOCAL PVC

24.SVT

25.VTACH

26.VTACH

27.AFIB

28.AFIB WITH ARTIFACT

29.AFLUTTER

30.SINUS WITH UNIFOCAL PVC

31.PACED

32.ATRIAL PACED

33.VFIB

34.SINUS BRADY WITH PVC

35.NSR

36.NSR WITH PVC

37.VTACH

38.BIGEMINY

39.SINUS BRADY

40."Q" WAVES & ELEVATED "T" WAVES (MI)

41.VFIB

42.VTACH

43.1ST DEGREE

44.SINUS WITH PVC

45.AFLUTTER

46.3RD DEGREE

47.AFIB

48.SVT

49.IDIOVENTRICULAR

50.3RD DEGREE

51.PACED

52.1ST DEGREE

53.ACCELERATED JUNCTIONAL

54.JUNCTIONAL

55.1ST DEGREE

56.2ND DEGREE

57.2ND DEGREE

58.2ND DEGREE

59.3RD DEGREE

60.SVT

61.AFIB

62.ASYSTOLE

63.TRIGEMINY

64.3RD DEGREE

65.AFLUTTER

66.AFIB

67.NSR WITH PVC

68.1ST DEGREE

69.AFIB

70.2ND DEGREE TYPE II

71.3RD DEGREE

72.BRADY

73.AFIB

74.VTACH

75.BRADY

>>

See Also:

12 Lead EKG…In about an hour!